High Praise for Mark Walters!

"Mark Walters shines a very bright light on the consequences of going unarmed in the United States."

– Kevin Michalowski
Executive Editor, *Concealed Carry* Magazine

"Mark Walters understands that guns are to self-defense as fire extinguishers are to fire safety. When Walters talks, smart people listen."

– Massad Ayoob
Author, *In the Gravest Extreme*

"Mark Walters is a great advocate of both defending your rights as well as your life. This book is a must read."

– Alan Gottlieb
Founder, Second Amendment Foundation

Hopefully "Lessons from Unarmed America" will awaken people to the need for awareness and preparedness before they become a victim. Hopefully "Lessons" will enable many of us to avoid dangerous pitfalls.

– Larry Pratt
Founder, Gun Owners of America

"Mark Walters and Rob Pincus are America's gun ownership champions. Their latest book, Lessons from Unarmed America is eye-opening proof that bad things happen to good people and that all of us should be ready to defend against the "wolves" who lurk among us."

– Scott Currie, Private Security Professional
Armed American Radio listener and I.C.E. Student

"Every week on national radio, Mark Walters tells listeners across the country to "never leave your cave without your club." In Lessons From Unarmed America, Mark and Rob remind us just how important that advice really is! This is required reading!"

– Sean C. "Seanto" Young
Executive Producer/Technical Director, Armed American Radio

"An exceptionally savvy addition to self-defense literature, these two experts have distilled the tactical essence that could spell the difference between life and death for you and your loved ones."

– Alan Korwin, Author of 10 books on American gun law

High Praise for Rob Pincus!

"Shemane and I learned much from Rob Pincus and respect him as one of the masters of the combat, self-defense training world."

– Ted Nugent
Rock-n-roll Legend
and author of *Ted, White and Blue*

"Rob Pincus is America's gunfighting coach. I have been a proponent of his training techniques for years and believe *Lessons from UNarmed America* is a must read for those learning about the consequences of choosing to be 'prey' in a world that continues to churn out 'predators.'"

– Kenneth R. Murray
Author, *Training at the Speed of Life*

"If you are reading this book, understand that Rob Pincus offers unique and brilliant perspective on everything he looks at, whether that be training, firearms, or any subject related. His dedication to researching the facts and basing his information on those findings, as well as being humble and intelligent enough to evolve as he learns more, make him an author and instructor that should be on anyones reading/training bucket list. There are many good gun and self defense books on the market, but if you desire a get to the point style with intelligent and unbiased lessons, the one you have in your hands is the one you should be reading right now!"

– Mike Seeklander
Owner, Shooting-Performance

Rob Pincus and Mark Walters are two of the great minds of our time. It has been my honor to count them both as friends and brother warriors. Separately they have made great contributions to our society. Together they have delivered an amazing book, that is essential reading for anyone who is interested in protecting themselves and their loved ones, in these violent times.

– Lt. Col. Dave Grossman,
Author of *On Combat* and *On Killing*

Published by White Feather Press, LLC
ISBN 978-1-61808-077-6

Printed in the United States of America

Cover design created by Betty Shonts

Disclaimer

The authors and publisher of this book assume that you, the reader, are an adult human being capable of making your own choices and taking responsibility for same. If you are not an adult, or are not capable of taking responsibility for your own choices, STOP. Do not read anything else in this book. The authors and publisher have made a reasonable, good-faith effort to assure that the book is accurate and contains good advice, but we hereby advise the reader that the authors and publisher are normal human beings who make the normal number of human mistakes. If something in this book sounds stupid or dangerous to you, don't do it. The authors and publisher accept absolutely no responsibility whatsoever for anything you might say or do as a result of reading any material in this book. Live your own life!

White Feather Press

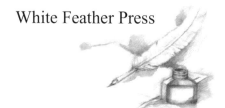

Reaffirming Faith in God, Family, and Country!

Contents

Chapter 1 - The Story of Oz.. 1

Chapter 2 - Dealing with Oz.. 11

Chapter 3 - Another Cold February Night 19

Chapter 4 - Dealing with Disarmament 29

Chapter 5 - I'm Always Aware of My Surroundings 35

Chapter 6 - Situational Awareness 43

Chapter 7 - Caroline and Rick Foster 49

Chapter 8 - Defending Against Stalkers........................... 59

Chapter 9 - The "Not So Restful" Stop............................ 81

Chapter 10 - The Problem: Isolation................................ 89

Chapter 11 - We Can Triumph Over Evil......................... 93

Chapter 12 - Domestic Violence 103

Chapter 13 - The Amanda Collins Story.......................... 109

Chapter 14 - Ambushed and Alone 119

Chapter 15 - In the Blink of an Eye 127

Chapter 16 - The Worst Moment 135

Mark's Final Thoughts... 140

Rob's Final Thoughts 142

Appendix I - School Shootings.. 147

Appendix II - Defensive Handgun Choice....................... 158

Lessons from UNarmed America

Mark Walters
&
Rob Pincus

Foreword
by Ted Nugent

Smart people admit unarmed helplessness is not only irresponsible, but, statistically, such carelessness is asking for trouble. Horrifically, I believe that a good guy who fails to stop a bad guy is complicit in the guaranteed next offense and victimization. It's supposed to be good over evil, not the other way around that the not-so-great society has so feebly embraced.

As the self-inflicted scourge of politically correct denial eats away at the American culture of rugged individualism and self-sufficiency, the brainwashing of dependency has turned otherwise decent human beings into sheep waiting to be had. If I hear another whiney voice feign shock over another rape, murder, assault, armed robbery, driveby shooting, kidnapping, dog attack, alligator attack, lion attack, bear attack, coyote attack, multi-paroled felon attack, repeat carjacking, monkey face-ripping attack or any number of virtually guaranteed life threatening incidents, I think I'm going to throw up.

You've got to be kidding me. Unarmed and helpless is not only wrong on every imaginable level, it is downright pathetic and embarrassing. We ask "how stupid can we get?" There is little in life more stupid than going about your daily life without any consideration for basic survival and fundamental preparedness, including carrying a gun, an adequate supply of ammo, and a proper understanding of the self-defense mindset and the proven tactics to go along with it all.

As I write this, Mrs. Nugent and I have just wrapped up another joyful fun day of tactical training 101 as the barrels on our rifles and handguns cool off. This is a regular regimen of enjoyable firearms activity that the Nugent family indulges in for all the right reasons. I have been a sworn sheriff deputy for more than 32 years and all of us have concealed carry permits and the powerful love of life and each other to inspire our capabilities and insistence to survive a deadly encounter. Plan B is for losers.

Shemane and I have had the distinct honor to train with the best of the best warriors. President GW Bush's personal counter-assault team trained and taught us on our SpiritWild Ranch in Texas, and we have burned up a lot of tax payer ammo with various SWAT, federal agencies, Navy SEALS, Army Rangers, and special ops, so we know how superior hard-core warriors can be. We are humbled by their dedication and talents and walk away each time further motivated to stand up against evil if and when it ever dares tread on us.

We've also had the distinct pleasure of training with Rob Pincus at a renowned facility a few years back, and believe that Rob is right up there with the best warriors. We learned much from Rob and respect him as one of the masters of the combat, self-defense training world.

When professionals like Mark Walters and Rob Pincus set out to write a book about the warrior spirit in contrast with the irresponsible condition and choice of helplessness, we can be assured there will be much enlightenment and guidance for those willing to stand and fight.

In this book, we get an overview of scenarios gone bad with life and death lessons on how to mitigate such conditions, and ultimately, how to be prepared so as to keep them from occurring in the first place.

The streets, hospitals, morgues and cemeteries are jam packed with the carcasses of losers who bought into the sheeping of America. It is always worth repeating that there have always been sheep, sheep dogs and wolves. Sadly, today in America there are more sheep than ever before, and the upgrade to sheepdog is not a difficult leap if one truly believes life is worth the effort.

Read this book carefully. Share it with your family, loved ones, friends and neighbors. It is time to reverse the constant slaughter of sheep and upgrade as many Americans as possible to be sheepdogs ready to neutralize the growing population of emboldened wolves out there, both literally and figuratively. Save the sheep, kill the wolves.

– Ted Nugent

Best-selling books
by Ted Nugent

God, Guns & Rock'N'Roll

Ted, White and Blue: The Nugent Manifesto

For more information on all things Ted Nugent, go to www.tednugent.com.

Preface

A word from the authors and publisher regarding the cowardly attack at the unarmed Sandy Hook Elementary School in Newtown, CT.

On December 14th, 2012 a crazed madman murdered his mother and subsequently attacked an unarmed and undefended elementary school in Newtown, CT., killing a total of 27 people in cold blood before sending himself to the gates of hell, hopefully to suffer and rot for all eternity. Included in that number are 20 first graders, 6 adult staff members and the attacker's mother. (We intentionally left out the murderer)

Although we briefly discuss the topic in this work, we felt it necessary to make this statement.

The authors and publisher of this book firmly and unequivocally believe that gun-free zones filled with unarmed potential victims present the greatest opportunities for killers to fulfill their goals of "scoring" high body counts. Virtually every mass shooting in America proves our point. Simply put, we believe that government sanctioned gun-free zones are in reality, killing zones and we can think of no better example of a crazed madman choosing a soft, unarmed, gun-free zone target than the Sandy Hook Elementary School.

According to the *N.Y. Daily News* and widely reported since (Lupica: Morbid find suggests murder obsessed gunman, Adam Lanza plotted Newtown Conn.'s Sandy Hook massacre for years, *NY Daily News*, published March 17th, 2013 and updated March 25th, 2013) during the International Association of Police Chiefs and Colonels mid-year meeting held in New Orleans in early March, 2013, CT. State Police Col. Danny Stebbins, spoke about the disturbing findings of a meticulous spreadsheet made by the CT. murderer. According to the report, "They believe that he picked an elementary school because he felt it was a point of least resistance, where he could rack up the greatest number of kills. That's what (the Connecticut State Police) believe."

We concur.

All of us (authors and publisher) are parents and there are simply no words to describe how we feel about what happened at Sandy Hook. Since then, author Rob Pincus has been teaching (free of charge) his School Attacker Response Course (SARC) to overflowing classrooms of parents and educators alike. Author and radio host Mark Walters continues to use Armed American Radio as a public platform to call for an end to phony "gun-free" school "safety zones". We believe it is insane to leave our most precious resources, our children, completely undefended and vulnerable to the next madman who ignores that "gun-free zone" sign.

For more information please visit:

www.schoolattackerresponse.com
www.armedamericanradio.com

First Introduction
By Mark Walters

I've often stated over the years that a criminal had a fifty-fifty shot at running into an armed victim if they chose me as their prey on any given day. That was before I made the decision to carry a firearm for personal protection everywhere I went as a result of an encounter on the streets of Tampa, Florida some years ago. (See Chapter 1, *Lessons from Armed America*, 2009 White Feather Press). I happened by chance to be armed that day. During that encounter I pulled my lawfully carried gun on two individuals to stop any potential further action against me. Yes, I had made the conscious decision to carry my gun that morning but only by chance. The odds that morning turned out in my favor, but may very well have favored the criminals had it been the day before. I can tell you with certainty that those odds are now 99% that a criminal will meet an armed victim if they choose me today. (The only thing keeping that number from being 100% would be if I find myself in an area that the law forbids me arming myself. That is rare, for I choose not to frequent those locations unless it is absolutely necessary).

There are anti-gunners or those who simply don't understand the right to bear arms that would call me paranoid for the statement I just made. I can assure you that couldn't be further from the truth for I choose not to frequent those places for the purpose of making a statement. For example, I will avoid a restaurant posted with a "No Guns Allowed" sign not out of fear of being unarmed while I eat, but rather I choose to put my wallet where my mouth is. As a public figure who loudly preaches the right to carry over the nation's airwaves, a "No Guns" sign equals no money for you if you blatantly ignore and deny my constitutional right to protect myself. Of course there is also the fact that as a result of what occurred several years ago, I choose not to be a victim. My firearm, coupled with my training over the years affords me the ability to defend myself … and that can only occur if my gun is with me.

One thing I have learned over many years is that life is not only about the choices we make but also about being prepared for the things we can not change. In order to be prepared we must first accept there are things we cannot change; there are things absolutely beyond our control and that evil does indeed exist. (Rob mentions this theme in his intro, and it also manifests itself throughout the stories you are about to read.) We literally must accept the fact that shit does indeed happen, and more than likely when we least expect it. Of course there are always exceptions. If you're gang banging on a drug-infested street corner then you might expect to become a victim of a drive-by, for example.

For most of us though I'm talking about the curveballs life inevitably throws at all of us at some point in our lives such as sickness requiring emergency medical care, a fall, a car wreck, fire, and, yes, even criminal attack. Only when we realize these things can and do occur when we least expect it, and accept it as part of life, can we begin the process of preparing for them when they take place. It's why we have insurance; it's why we teach children to stop, drop and roll, or why we have storm safety drills in schools, etc. The problem we face as human beings is we would rather not think of these things happening to us, which makes it easy for us to ignore the facts, thereby making us even more vulnerable when something does happen. And guess what? Something will happen someday, and those who survive will more than likely be those who are prepared.

While the premise of this work focuses on being unarmed during a violent or potentially violent encounter, it is also to remind you that being unarmed does not always mean being without a physical tool such as a firearm. No, being unarmed can also mean simply being unprepared for the pitfalls of life as we go through our normal, busy day. You'll read the story of my son choking on a street corner after dinner, and I'll explain my immediate response to that frightening occurrence. Clearly, that wasn't a situation requiring my use of a firearm; however, it did require being armed with another tool: knowledge. I was armed with the knowledge necessary to save my little guy and was prepared to use that knowledge when it mattered most, thank God. Another story from my own life experiences will teach you to trust your gut instincts, for they are usually always right. You'll read about violent criminal attacks and learn from the responses of others as they found their lives on the line, literally.

Continuing in the groundbreaking format of *Lessons from Armed America*, co-written with Kathy Jackson, this work brings the story to life and follows it with analysis from Rob Pincus. You'll read invaluable commentary from one of the best personal defense instructors in the world. You will learn from the experiences of others and, with the benefit of hindsight and many years of study and experience, the lessons you take away from this work may one day save your life.

Second Introduction
by Rob Pincus

Evil Exists.
You may be visited by Evil.
You should be prepared to Defend Yourself against that Evil.

To me, those statements are all self-evident. Many people in our world don't seem to agree. The fact that you are reading this book indicates that you may be inclined to agree with my way of thinking. If you aren't, the stories in this book may convince you that you should. It is necessary that you take that step before my contributions to this work can truly be valuable to you. Without a keen understanding of the three simple sentences at the top of this page, all the good advice in the world about how to deal with an unexpected attack may do you no good at all when you need it.

Overwhelmingly, people who are visited by evil will tell you that they "couldn't believe" it was happening or they "never imagined" it would happen to them or at the place that it did. Let the stories in this book be a testament to the fact that the existence of the unexpected attack is exactly what you need to accept. I refer to the style of personal defense that I teach as *counter ambush*, because that is exactly what you are going to need to do in the worst-case personal defense scenario: counter an ambush that is being brought down on you. There will be no time to plan, little time to make decisions and there is not likely to be time for a detailed analysis of options. Planning ahead to respond in specific ways to specific attacks, to behave in certain ways in certain situations and to take action in the face of attack is the best thing you can do. Even if you take none of the specific advice I offer in this book, please take this paragraph to heart. By the very definition, you will *not* be ready for an ambush. If you are going to take the time to plan to defend yourself or your family, please do not limit yourself to only preparing for threats that you see coming… those are the easy fights.

When Mark Walters invited me to join this project, I was very excited about it. The groundwork for the format that Mark Walters and Kathy Jackson laid down in *Lessons from Armed America* is a great one for both teaching and learning. Humans are storytellers. Everyone loves a good story, and the best ones can serve as examples through which we can learn and memory anchors that bring emotion to the, sometimes dry and technical, process of learning. For someone whose writing is generally without much to offer in terms of engaging story arcs, this type of work is a nice change.

There is, however, an intimidating twist to working with these stories: They are true stories about real people. In order to do my job, I was going to have to point out things that were done that I wouldn't advise. No matter how we couch the language, my role here in many cases is to point out *mistakes* that were made by people who have already suffered and are often looked upon as heroes by those who know them and their stories. What did they do that I would suggest you *not* do? What would I suggest you do, which they *neglected* to do? Only by "Monday Morning Quarterbacking" their stories, can I hope to offer important insight and valuable ideas to you.

It is important to note that this is done with all due respect and a great appreciation for the people whose lives we are hoping to learn from. Too often, people shy away from critiquing actions after a violent attack. Out of sympathy for what the victims of violence have already been through and out of a sincere respect for the fact that they survived, despite possible mistakes, many people defer to saying things like "whatever works, works" or "you can't blame the victim". Yes, ultimately it is true that we would never want someone to lose a fight instead of winning it "wrongly" and the person ultimately responsible for violence is the perpetrator, not the victim.

That said, I would much rather that *you* make choices and take actions that might prevent you from finding yourself in some of the situations you are about to read about. In some cases, I would much rather that *you* make *different* choices and take *better* actions. By critiquing and learning from these stories, we can make people safer … and, I believe that the people who play the starring roles in what you are about to read would be pleased with that. As you read this book, remember that the people you are about to read about were operating without the benefit of hindsight. They were also operating without the benefit of the advice you are about to read.

When I've talked to people who have been visited by evil, they have almost always stated that they could've altered one or two things about the days, hours or moments leading up to their incident that would've changed things dramatically. In many cases, those simple alterations would've meant that there was no incident at all. As you read this, you are days, hours or moments away from making a decision that could save your life.

I hope you find this work useful in your planning process and your preparation to defend yourself against evil. Evil *does* exist and you may be visited by it.

Train Well!

Lessons from UNarmed America

by
Mark Walters
&
Rob Pincus

This book is dedicated to every victim, every state and national grassroots group and its members and all those fighting for the right to bear arms against the individuals and freedom-hating groups who would blame an inanimate object for the actions of criminals. Those same people who see the firearm as a tool of evil rather than one used thousands of times every day by good law-abiding, hard-working people to defend themselves from evil predators. This work is dedicated to American gun owners who refuse to be intimidated by them. To the tireless individuals everywhere fighting those sanctimonious individuals who make it their life's work to strip freedom from the constitution with their daily attacks against our sacred second amendment right to bear arms. To those sleeping with toothpicks under their eyes while the sheep sleep soundly in their beds at night, this work is dedicated to each of you.

The Story

There is an aspect of self-defense that has nothing to do with firearms, but is every bit as crucial if you are to survive a life-threatening encounter. This story is an important reminder of that life lesson.

Chapter 1 - The Story of Oz

Mark Walters

As the introduction pointed out, not all of the encounters written about in this book are of violent crimes, but every one of them can be considered an individual lesson. Such is the case with Oz, a personal story from my own life that stands as a stark and disturbing reminder that the things we take for granted and the people we meet as we wend through life aren't always who they appear to be. The lessons learned from Oz are important for all of us, both in and out of the workplace.

During the mid-nineties I had left the security of my corporate job to start a business of my own. It had always been a dream of mine to be in business for myself, working on my own, not having to answer to anyone, thereby allowing me the prospect of enjoying the fruits of my own hard work or deal with the failures of my shortcomings. I was willing to find out which it would be. That opportunity would present itself to me shortly after moving to Tampa, Florida.

As a sales representative for a large trucking company, I had daily contact with many industrial customers who needed help reducing their transportation budgets. I had recognized early in my career that there might be occasion for me to help these businesses on my own in ways the trucking companies weren't. It frustrated me to see so many firms spending far more than was necessary on transportation costs, and I often wondered what the owners would do if they were aware of the wasteful spending occurring right under their noses. My desire to do something about it peaked when I walked through the doors of a growing snack food manufacturing company in Ft. Myers.

During a prescheduled appointment to discuss their transportation needs, I was shocked when, without hesitation and without listening to one word that I had to say, the traffic manager and owners offered me their business with no knowledge whatsoever of my prices as long as I "matched the current discount" given by my competitors. They meant no harm to themselves; they just didn't understand the intricacies of the freight world. They were a small company beginning to move a substantial amount of product, and their freight costs might literally determine their survival if they weren't careful. These were good people, and I felt an innate desire to help them. I seized the opportunity to explain to them what they had just done, offered them my assistance "on the side" to analyze and reduce their expenses, and I walked out with a $3,000 retainer check for my consulting services with agreement to accept a percentage of the future savings I created as contracted payment. In other words, I saved them money or I made nothing.

I was in business! The opportunity was upon me, and I used that as my inspiration to "jump ship." What started out as a simple freight consulting business eventually blossomed into a much bigger endeavor. Before I knew it, I had taken on two partners and was running a more complex venture than I had originally anticipated, quickly morphing the consulting business into an operation offering a full range of trucking services.

I met one of my partners through my previous employer when he was transferred to my office in Tampa. It was my responsibility to show Kent the ropes in his new sales territory. Right away, we seemed to hit it off well on a personal level. As I had gotten to know him a little better over many months of working together, I developed a sense of trust in him. I mentioned what I had planned and asked if he was interested in quitting his job to help me run the consulting company. He agreed.

Our other partner was a close friend of mine whom I had met through mutual acquaintances shortly after relocating to Tampa and long before I had met Kent. He and his family owned a large and well-respected insurance brokerage business in town as well as the office building in which the company was located. He and his father provided us the office space to launch our consulting and brokerage firm. I was scared, nervous, and excited about my future and what lay ahead.

Like all small business owners who take a risk, we took whatever steps we felt necessary to ensure the success of our start-up operation. Kent moved into my two-bedroom apartment in a "not so nice" area of town to share expenses. We pooled what little money we had to live off of until we could grow a customer base and we worked like dogs. Twenty-hour workdays were not unheard of as we were getting ourselves off of the ground. With persistence and hard work, we had begun to create a small customer base that was finally creating an income stream, limited as it was.

It soon became apparent that we needed help, and the decision was made to bring on a sales person. We figured we could try to build a customer base faster if we had some "boots on the ground" while the two of us did the required customer service and consulting work which was the core of the business. It worked. Soon we had some commissioned sales help that didn't cost a fortune, and the two of us were able to man the phones and do the inside heavy lifting.

As time progressed, the company continued to evolve almost on its own. Unfortunately, my business relationship with Kent was beginning to deteriorate. Our visions changed; he had met a young lady and had begun putting less effort into the business, choosing instead to focus more on his personal life. After much soul-searching and lengthy discussions with my other partner, we were duty-bound to relieve Kent of his ownership stake in the business. It was a tough call, but for the sake of the future of my fledgling company, it was the right one. Kent's contract was immediately terminated and he and his girlfriend would soon leave Tampa to start a new life together in the greater Atlanta area.

With the passage of time, no more partner problems, and an increasing customer base came more success and growth opportunity. I soon had another new sales representative and agreed to hire an additional staff member to support his sales effort.

I had met Osborne, or Oz as we called him, several months earlier at a local restaurant and gathering place many of us regularly frequented after work in the Tampa Palms area of the city. Oz was there after work every day enjoying a glass of scotch and eating hot wings. I had struck up conversation with him on many occasions and found him to be an incredibly engaging individual. He was a nice man, well dressed and soft spoken with what sounded like an island-flavored accent. I would later find out he had family roots in Kenya, and with the exception of his wife, he had no family here in America. Oz had an incredibly unique personality with a distinctive character and charisma that I had rarely seen. He got along well with all of the other regular patrons, and I enjoyed his company as we discussed life in general, his wife, and other normal small talk. That small talk would eventually become discussions about his disdain for his current employer and his ongoing search for a new job. Oz had heard from others that I was looking for some help, and eventually approached me about the possibility of joining my company.

He had no background in my industry, but he sure could get a conversation started. He was easy to talk to, and his engaging personality made me believe that if properly trained, he would be an incredible asset.

I hired him.

Just as I had thought, Oz's unique character and his flair for conversation were an instant hit with the customers. He enjoyed his job and told me on more than one occasion that he felt relief from the pressure he was under from his former employer. He seemed happy and "life was good," as he used to say.

Not long after beginning his employment with my company, my partner had agreed to hire Oz's wife, Andrea. Soft spoken and very pretty, Andrea went to work in the customer service department of his family's insurance brokerage firm in the same building. Like Oz, she was very well liked by all of the employees and had an excellent work ethic.

Oz and Andrea would arrive to work on time, leave together for lunch each day, return punctually and leave together in the afternoon. It seemed like a perfect match, however, things would soon begin to change. As Oz became more comfortable around me, I noticed subtle transformations in his behavior. Always punctual in the mornings at the start of a work day, he began to disappear for lengthy durations during the day at off times, leaving to go pay a bill or head over to the local convenience store. The excuses began to pile up. When confronted about the random breaks, he would become agitated, roll his eyes or make a snarky comment. He would compare his behavior to other employees with a childlike attitude of, "I bet it would be okay if Jim did it," for example.

As time passed his erratic behavior became an increasing concern, both in and out of the office. Having been given a speeding ticket in a residential neighborhood near the building on his way into work one morning, Oz entered the office irate. Blaming the police officer for giving him the ticket because he "was black," he vowed to fight it in court on racial grounds. He was becoming irritated more easily and seemed to have lost much of the fun and unique character that drew me to him in the first place.

As a business owner, the possibility of workplace violence was never far from my mind. As much as I tried not to think about it, I couldn't disregard the possibility. I began to keep a more watchful eye on Oz from a safety standpoint, because he was beginning to make others in the building uncomfortable.

His bizarre transformation continued. He began asking my other employees for money, claiming that things were "tight" and that he needed some financial help. Eventually he turned to me with the same requests. He soon began asking me for loans, telling me he was "short" that week, had "bills to pay," and was sick of "living in the 'shithole" he shared with his wife. (Oz and his wife lived in a run-down little apartment complex in a seedy little area of North Tampa.) He would tell me in an angry manner that he was "just trying to make a better life for his lady." I felt sorry for him, but refused to *lend* him any money over and above his base pay and his commissions. He knew that the key to his success was hard work, equaling higher commission payments.

Over the next few days and weeks, it became apparent that Oz wasn't going to make it. I was getting uncomfortable around him. My partner was uncomfortable. He was making others in the building nervous and, quite frankly, he just wasn't acting right. I was unable to deduce exactly what was happening, but it was obvious that his behavior was changing for the worse. The charisma he exuded when we had first met was disappearing by the day.

Regrettably, I had no other option but to terminate him. It was a tough decision; I mean I liked the guy! I didn't appreciate being put in this position, and I was upset that things turned out the way they had as I had always enjoyed his company both personally and professionally. Despite that, I had to worry about the safety and security of my other employees.

Surprisingly, Oz went without an argument. When terminated, he quietly packed his belongings from the desk, walked down the hall, told his wife to gather her things, informed her she no longer worked there and I watched as the two of them quietly left the building together. Although I never saw them again, I did find out from a mutual industry contact that he had left Florida and was still working within the transportation industry somewhere in the Carolinas. I admit that I felt a sense of pride that he had learned enough from me to at least be able to seek employment within the field I had taught him.

Two years had passed when a young lady who had befriended Andrea during her tenure at the insurance company walked into my office. She proceeded to tell me the story about a phone call she had just received from someone claiming to be the sister of Oz's wife. I listened intently as the truth about Oz and his wife unfolded before me. My eyes closed and I took a deep breath when I heard that he was being held in the Lowndes County Jail near Valdosta, Georgia, awaiting trial on charges of murder and possession of a firearm during the commission of a crime.

Oz had been arrested for murdering his wife. After spending nearly two years behind bars in the Lowndes County Jail awaiting trial, he plead guilty to voluntary manslaughter. He is currently serving a mandatory 20 years with no possibility of parole, and, as of this writing is doing his time in a Georgia State penitentiary approximately 125 miles south of Atlanta. He will be 70 years old when he is eventually released from his sentence in 2022.

Another sad note: I lost touch with my former business partner, Kent, shortly after he was released from his contract. After relocating to the greater metropolitan Atlanta area myself, we had begun rekindling our friendship over the next year and a half. We had agreed to meet in early December 2007 before everyone became too busy during the Christmas season. After several unsuccessful attempts to reach him by cell phone to confirm the date and time, I gave up and never heard from him again. Two years later I would find out that he had been found dead on the kitchen floor of his suburban Atlanta home on Saturday, December 8, 2007, from a stab wound... the very week we were to have gotten together. My heart sank as I read the details of his wife being arrested and charged with his murder. After spending two years in the Gwinnett County Jail awaiting trial for the death of her husband, she was eventually acquitted of all charges in January 2010 by a jury of her peers. The mystery surrounding his death remains officially unsolved.

Life-saving tip

Always listen to that little voice inside your head that sometimes notices when things are wrong long before you have overt "proof".

Chapter 2 - Dealing with Oz

Rob Pincus

The Problem:

PEOPLE NATURALLY WANT TO TRUST OTHERS. MOST HUMAN beings seek out interaction, partnership and tend to naturally give others the benefit of the doubt. While it usually means cooperation and mutual success, this trait can be a fatal flaw when it comes up against someone who isn't capable of abiding by the same social contract. If someone is one of the wolves that roam our society looking for victims, they will betray that trust.

The safety net that we have to protect us from blindly trusting others is our intuition. Our intuition, in this sense, is comprised of many inarticulable "gut feelings". These non-cognitive decisions that we make based on subtle observations, prejudices, experiences and the behavior of others can literally save our lives … if we listen to them.

In Mark's start-up business, we see examples of this safety net both working and failing. First, we can look at the decision to let Oz go as an example of Mark trusting his intuition and deciding to distance himself from this person. Next, we have both Oz's wife and Kent who both actually lived with people who were eventually charged with murder and yet didn't take action to separate themselves from them. While it is certainly possible that someone would "snap" and instantly commit a violent crime with no precursor actions at all (and that may have been the case with Kent's wife) the fact that Mark had bad feelings about Oz indicates that his wife, for some reason, didn't see or chose to ignore those precursors. Here's another possibility. Because Kent's wife was acquitted of all charges, it is possible there were circumstances of violence *against* her in the home and that Kent's killing was justified as an act of self-defense in the mind of the jury.

> It isn't easy to stop trusting someone in a close personal relationship.

Another issue that we must address is that Mark's decision to terminate his relationship with Oz was made in a business environment. Naturally, it is going to be easier to stop trusting someone in a professional capacity than it is inside a personal relationship. Overwhelmingly, acts of violence in our society, especially against women, happen at the hands of people who were known and trusted by the victim prior to the attack. Whether it is a romantic relationship, a family member or a trusted person in your community, betrayal of that trust

12

needs to remain a possibility in our minds at all times. This doesn't mean having impenetrable walls that keep you from having relationships; it simply means keeping your guard up and being open to suggestions from that little voice inside your head that sometimes notices when things are wrong long before we have overt "proof".

Ultimately, this entire drama is a stark reminder that danger is all around us, and we must not only be wary and on the lookout for overt warning signs, but also that we shouldn't second-guess our own intuitive internal warning system.

Change the Story:

IMAGINE FOR A MOMENT THAT MARK HAD DECIDED TO TALK TO Andrea about Oz's behavior change prior to terminating him. The conversation might have resulted in Andrea thinking harder about whether or not she wanted to trust Oz. Perhaps the conversation would've resulted in her confronting Oz and pushing him to seek help for his anger and frustration. Maybe, it would have set Oz off on a violent rampage in the work place. The many variables are what make these situations so hard to

> **People want to trust others. They seek out partnership and friendship.**

deal with in our society. Of course, there is also the reality of the "it's none of my business" attitude that most people feel very comfortable taking in these situations.

It is hard to argue that Mark's action (distancing himself and his business from someone with deviant and erratic behavior) wasn't the *right* thing to do to protect himself. It's possible that confronting Oz more directly by speaking to Andrea or bringing Oz's potentially violent nature to the attention of the authorities could actually have escalated the situation.

When people step outside of what is commonly seen as their area of "responsibility", they are sometimes themselves ostracized. Unfortunately, it has become part of the accepted social contract to distance one's self from actions that might actually protect others who won't act for themselves. If we want to make society safer, we might need to take an extra step from time to time. However, extreme care should be taken as this is a very fine line, and one that must be crossed delicately when you simply have a "bad feeling" about a person but nothing overt to act on.

> Sometime we might need to take an additional step to help protect other innocent people.

Preparation and Training:

LEARNING TO TRUST THAT LITTLE VOICE INSIDE YOUR HEAD CAN be emotionally uncomfortable. Talking to people about your feelings is something that, especially for men, can create awkward social pressures. Taking actions and making decisions in life that you cannot incontrovertibly justify to others who don't have your same intuitive feelings is often difficult. Most people avoid those situations when they can.

Learning to embrace that awkwardness and to deal with confrontations over intuition can happen at low levels in your everyday life. Simply asserting non-conformity in your relationships and your peer groups can make you much more comfortable with trusting your own intuition.

> **Learn to trust that little voice inside your head that makes you feel uncomfortable.**

For example, be willing to voice your opinion when a group of friends or co-workers decides where to go for dinner and the group decision doesn't sit well with you. Don't be afraid to go against the consensus. Too often, people just "go with the flow" and don't act on their own feelings for the sake of avoiding even very low levels of confrontation. For many people, this habit of minimizing the value of their own comfort for the sake of other individuals or the group can lead to a paralyzing inability to act that actually puts them in danger when the boyfriend, co-worker or family member begins to take advantage of their non-confrontational nature.

> **Human predators look for people who trust too quickly and easily.**

Some predators in our society look for people who don't know how to *distrust* or are uncomfortable with challenging those who would try to manipulate them. We need to be prepared to make hard decisions, voice opinions that could cause conflict and to take actions that go against the status-quo in our relationships. You might even find situations where you can put a toe over the line into something that society might say "doesn't concern you" and find yourself in a position to help someone else avoid becoming a victim of someone that they trust a little too much.

This is a touchy area when it comes to personal defense. Strictly speaking, you have done your job by separating yourself from the person that you feel could be a problem. By crossing that line and getting involved to protect others, you *may* be putting yourself in more danger. Again, this is a place where you trust your intuition and do what you feel is right.

Be careful who you let into your life

- According to the National Institute of Justice about 85 to 90 percent of sexual assaults reported by college women are perpetrated by someone known to the victim; about half occur on a date. The most common locations are the man's or woman's home in the context of a party or a date. The perpetrators may range from classmates to neighbors.

- Based on data from the FBI's Supplementary Homicide Reports (SHR) strangers committed between 21 percent and 27 percent of homicides while between 73 percent and 79 percent of murderers knew their victims. This tells us that most often murder victims are killed for a specific reason. Most often the murderer is acquainted with the victim, and attacked them out of anger, envy, lust, greed, or for some other personal reason. It is more unusual for a stranger to murder another stranger.

- According to Cathy Steinberg, in her book *The Fabulous Girl's Guide to Being Fearless*, murderers and rapists exist and are counting on your trusting, compassionate nature to harm you.

"Only two steps and I heard somebody say something. I turned around and looked back and asked what they had said when I saw the passenger behind the driver in the back seat was pointing a gun at me."

Chapter 3 - Another Cold February Night

Mark Walters

LIKE 7,000 OTHER GEORGIA RESIDENTS, I AM A PROUD member of Georgiacarry.org (GCO), the state's pre-eminent grassroots Second Amendment organization. I'm proud to say that I am one of the first 800 members or there-abouts, according to past president Ed Stone. The nation's state-level grassroots organizations provide an opportunity for residents like you and I to get involved in the policies that impact our right to carry a firearm and defend ourselves and our families in our home states regardless of where we live. In the few short years since I have lived in Georgia for example, I can say with certainty that Georgia's carry laws are now far less restrictive than my adopted home state of Florida's as a direct result of GCO's tireless activism during the time I have been here. With the exception of the change in Georgia law removing the 150-year-old restriction on carrying a firearm at a "public gathering," none of those changes had been more profound than the passage of legislation allowing law-abiding firearms license holders to carry their firearms in restaurants and establishments that serve alcohol.

In addition to having an impact on state law, the grass-roots organizations also provide an opportunity for folks to meet other like-minded members who are concerned about the erosion of our freedoms, particularly with regard to our Second Amendment. In an effort to foster this camaraderie, GCO hosts an annual meeting and convention which provides all of the members from across the state the opportunity to meet with other members, the board of directors, and special guests. It was at just one of these meetings (the 3rd annual Georgia Carry convention to be exact) where I had a booth set up next to one of my personal heroes, Ms. Suzanna Gratia Hupp.

Ms. Hupp was inside the Luby's Cafeteria in Killeen, Texas on October 16, 1991 having lunch with her parents and a friend when maniac George Hennard drove his truck through the plate glass window and into the crowded restaurant, exited his vehicle, and began systematically and methodically shooting the diners. Ms. Hupp watched in horror as her father rushed the murderer in a desperate, but vain attempt to stop the carnage, only to be shot in the chest, the projectile piercing his heart. Her mother, who had rushed to his side during the ongoing rampage, cradled her dying husband's head in her lap and looked up to find the madman standing directly before her. The two made eye contact and in front of the Hupp's daughter, Suzanna, George Hennard leveled his handgun directly at her mother and fired, killing her instantly. When the smoke had cleared, 23 innocent patrons lay dead or dying, including Ms. Hupp's mother and father.

Suzanna Hupp escaped that day and went on to become a Texas state legislator, fighting for the right to keep and bear arms. Like her on that fateful day, six other patrons were following Texas state law that forbids them from carrying their lawful handguns into the restaurant. As a result, the psychopath was able to continue the killing unabated until police arrived.

Her story is well known and no matter how many times I hear her tell it, I am moved beyond words, particularly when she is standing directly in front of me. On this August day, the two of us were meeting with GCO members and selling our books alongside other vendors ranging from firearms dealers to jewelry makers. Suzanna was in town as the keynote speaker at the dinner function scheduled for later that evening.

Next to us was a table manned by GCO volunteers who travel throughout the state signing up new members at gun shows, stores, and events, etc. Member Dan Agrimonte whom I had met through the organization on previous occasions and another member, "Buddy," staffed this particular booth. All of us chatted about the event and listened intently to Dr. Hupp tell her story. Like the rest of us, Buddy was engaged in the conversation with Dan and I as we listened to her.

Later, I noticed Buddy was engaged in a private conversation with Ms. Hupp who was listening intently. I could tell by her expressions that this was a story I too wanted to hear. Turning toward me after he finished his conversation, he mentioned to me that he was a fan of the Armed American Radio show and proceeded to tell me his own story of being robbed at gunpoint, the same story he had told Ms. Hupp just moments earlier. As is always the case, I was captivated by the intensity of his story and, like Suzanna, sat listening fixedly. I immediately asked his permission to write about it. He gladly obliged and we promised to get together soon. Of course time flies and it wasn't until we met at the following year's convention that we finally got around to making it happen. What you are about to read are the events that unfolded on a freezing, early February 2000 night in the northern suburbs of Atlanta. It was a night that would almost cost GCO member Buddy his life.

Marietta Georgia – Friday, February 5, 2000

"IT WAS COLD, MAN. I REMEMBER HOW COLD IT WAS," 32-YEAR-old Buddy recalled. Anyone familiar with the Atlanta area summers knows that they're long, hot, and muggy. The Fall brings a crisp and chilly relief from the heat and although not known as a cold weather city, the metropolitan Atlanta area can get downright nasty cold in the midst of the wintertime. Such was the case on Friday, February 5th, 2000 and the weather mattered to Buddy. A landscaper, Buddy and his crews would spend all day outside in the winter cold looking forward to knocking off for a warm shower, a change of clothes, and on Fridays some camaraderie after work at the local Mexican restaurant off of Rt. 41 in Marietta, Georgia, which they regularly frequented together as a large group of twenty-five friends.

Buddy arrived at the restaurant at about 7:30 p.m. as customary. A long-time licensed Georgia firearm permit holder, he removed his lawfully carried Taurus PT 945 from his holster and locked the gun inside his truck's glove box, following Georgia law at the time which forbade the carrying of a firearm inside a restaurant,. Heading inside, Buddy and his friends enjoyed their regular Friday festivities of good food, drink, and conversation. Winding down at about 9:30 p.m. a young lady friend, another regular group member, told him she was getting, "kind of bored" and asked Buddy if he felt like heading down the road to a local country western club.

"We got there; we hung out for a little while. She was just an acquaintance and I got bored after a while and was ready to go. She didn't want to go and since she drove, I went to the front and asked the guy at the door to call me a cab to get back to my truck," Buddy recalled. The Mexican restaurant was only about three miles down the road. Buddy stepped outside into the cold and waited for the cab for "over an hour and a half," he remembered. "It was about 12:30 a.m. and I was about to freeze to death, so I went back inside and asked the guy to call the cab back. It never showed up. I just got sick of waiting and decided I was going to walk back to the truck."

Buddy figured that for as long as he had stood outside freezing near to death he could have walked back and been in his truck already. Taking off from the club, he began the approximately three-mile trek down US 41 Cobb Parkway to get back to his vehicle. "I'd been walking twenty, maybe thirty minutes or so when a car stopped. Inside there were five black teenage males. They asked me where I was going and if I needed a ride. I told them I was going up the road to the Mexican restaurant and they told me they needed gas money."

"You give us some gas money and we'll give you a ride." one of the passengers yelled to Buddy out the window.

"Sounds like a plan to me! Will ten bucks work then?" he asked them.

"That'd be great," they told him. "Hop in." Buddy jumped in the back seat, grateful for the short ride a mile or so up the road and thankful he was out of the cold.

"The Mexican restaurant was at the corner of U.S. Hwy 41 and Bells Ferry Road and they passed it," he said. Letting them know they had passed his destination, they stopped immediately at the Waffle House "right next door," near the corner of the side of the building only "six feet or so" from the building itself.

"They were just typical teenagers, dressed in jeans and sweatshirts on a cold night," Buddy remembered. "There was nothing at the time that made me concerned," he said. No red flags had gone up during the short ride as Buddy remembered there was nothing but typical small talk. Not thinking anything was amiss when the car stopped, he exited the rear passenger seat and walked up to the passenger side front window. Reaching into his wallet, he pulled out the agreed upon ten dollars for the ride, thanked the young guys who had saved him from the remainder of his cold walk, handed it to the front seat passenger through the open window and turned toward the rear of the car to walk next door to his truck.

"There were two kids in the front seat and three in the back seat," Buddy said. As he stepped away from the car he recalled, "Only two steps and I heard somebody say something. I turned around and looked back and asked what they had said when I saw the passenger behind the driver in the back seat was pointing a gun at me."

Pointing the gun directly at him and reaching over the two other back-seat passengers, he yelled through the open window for Buddy to give him his wallet. "I pulled all of the other money I had out of my wallet which was only about thirty or forty dollars and the front seat passenger took the rest of the cash. He then told me he *wanted* my wallet. That's when I turned and ran," Buddy said.

Taking off alongside the stopped car toward the safety of the entrance to the Waffle House a mere six feet away, wallet in hand, he heard the crack of the gunshot that hit him. "As I was rounding the corner I heard the gunshot. I felt what felt like a cross between a bee sting and tetanus shot," he said, "a burning sensation in my buttocks and hip area ... upper area near my hip. I continued to run until I came around to the front door. I went into the Waffle House and there were three employees and a customer in there. I said, 'I've been shot, please dial 911.' and the cook was already on the phone with the 911 operator, having heard the gunshot and dialed 911."

Coming to his aid immediately, one of the waitresses tried to calm him and get him to sit down. "One of the waitresses came around the corner trying to keep pressure on it," he said referring to his wound. Still standing, Buddy wasn't about to sit down. "These guys are still out there, take cover, I don't know where they're at and I don't know what's going on!" he said to the staff. "While all this is going on, the car comes around to the front of the Waffle House to the road and has to stop because a car is coming. The traffic delayed them long enough that the cook was able to grab the license number and give it to the Marietta police when they got there." he said.

Bleeding profusely, shot in the upper right buttocks/hip area, the waitress finally convinced Buddy to sit down until help arrived. Agreeing, he sat uncomfortable at the edge of one of the booths. The police and ambulance crews arrived quickly, "within a couple of minutes," Buddy said, "They cut all of my clothes away and laid me on the stretcher," for the short ride to the local hospital.

After spending several hours at Wellstar Kennestone Hospital, Buddy was released and recovered completely from the injuries sustained during the armed robbery. The robbers, five teenagers all related and ranging in age from 15-19 years old were caught by Marietta police attempting to flee the area within minutes of the robbery and shooting. "They were from Greenville, South Carolina or something like that and were in the area visiting relatives. One of them was from the area here," Buddy recalled. Two guns were found inside the vehicle. Four of the criminals plead guilty and received a one-year sentence each for their crimes, receiving the time served while awaiting a trial. The shooter, the front seat passenger, and the oldest of the bunch at 19-years-old refused a plea agreement and decided to stand trial. As a result of his failure to plead guilty and his decision to try the case, he was convicted in November 2001 and received a 30-year sentence for aggravated battery. Although he will be eligible for parole, at the time this goes to press he is still incarcerated.

Like Texas law had done to Ms. Hupp and several other diners that day in Texas years earlier, Georgia law disarmed Buddy. At the time of his robbery, it was illegal for a concealed carry permit holder to enter a restaurant or establishment that served alcohol. That law has since been changed in both states.

Questions about pistol-free zones

PISTOL-FREE ZONES, OFTEN CALLED "CRIMINAL SAFE ZONES" OR "criminal empowerment zones" by the pro-gun community, vary from state to state. When comparing the different lists from across the states, they seem to make very little sense.

For example:
- In North Carolina it's illegal to carry concealed in a funeral procession.
- In Tennessee guns are not allowed in the state capitol.
- In Michigan both pistols and long guns are allowed in the state capitol for both concealed and open carry.
- However, in Michigan it's illegal to carry in a daycare center or a sports stadium. Go figure.
- What is it that makes North Carolina residents untrustworthy at a funeral?
- Why can Michigan residents be trusted in their state capitol while Tennesseans cannot?
- Why can Tennesseans carry in a bar while the residents of most other states are prohibited? Is it something in the water? Is it better whiskey?

One things is certain, the levying of pistol-free zones seems to be illogical and capricious. What were those lawmakers thinking?

A firearm is not a magic talisman of safety any more than it is a menace to society.

Chapter 4 - Dealing with Disarmament

Rob Pincus

The Problem:

BY NOW, YOU CAN PROBABLY PREDICT THE BIGGEST MIStakes that Buddy made that night: Isolation and misplaced trust. These recurring themes are important and you should be able to easily identify how Buddy could've avoided being in the situation he was in …. probably at every step: staying out late in an unknown area, separating from friends, hitchhiking.

Too often, people believe that if they were able to simply carry a gun, they would be safer. Unfortunately, that is simply not true. A firearm is not a magic talisman of safety any more than it is a menace to society. As we so often want to remind those who are anti-gun, the firearm is just a tool … an inanimate object that can do nothing without an operator. That operator chooses how to store and use the firearm. The operator can make good decisions or bad, be a person with the best intentions or the worst.

Change the Story:

THERE ARE A FEW EASY DECISIONS THAT COULD'VE MADE THE night go dramatically differently. It is also easy to see how a few of those decisions (not going out with friends, not splitting up the group, etc.) would've resulted in Buddy actually changing from the course of action that he wanted to follow. It is important to note, however, that you may not have to radically alter your lifestyle or behavior choices in order to improve your safety. If Buddy had not given up control of his own transportation, he would never have been walking on the side of the road. That decision alone is the one that would've had no negative impact on anything else Buddy did, but would most certainly have kept him from needing a cab, standing outside for a ridiculous amount of time, deciding to walk back to his car and, most importantly, getting into that car on the side of the road.

> Don't go to places you don't know or don't feel comfortable.

Maintaining control of your location, communication and transportation options is an easy way to be able to decrease your likelihood of being put at risk because of the actions of others. Don't go to places you don't know or don't feel comfortable, maintain your ability to communicate with others (i.e., have a cell phone and have it charged!) and, whenever possible, hold the keys (literally and/or figuratively) to your own ability to leave a location when you decide to.

In the exact moment of conflict, with a gun pointed at him, Buddy could also have chosen to hand over his wallet. Far more people are robbed at the *threat* of a lethal attack than are actually the victims of a lethal attack. We can't second-guess someone's intuition, but we should remember that the loss or destruction of property is not worth causing a situation to become one that could kill you.

> Buddy could also have chosen to hand over his wallet.

It is very hard to predict the actions of a criminal (already deviant, by definition), but be sure to keep "cooperating until…" as an option in your mind.

The last change we can discuss is the option of having a firearm. If Buddy *had* the option to carry a firearm legally and chosen to take it, the situation he was in may not have been any different. When confronted with a gun pointed at you without warning, it may be too late to draw your own gun. Unlike the situation that Suzanna was in that tragic day in the restaurant, there was no moment described in Buddy's event where he could've taken time to draw his firearm and not been in immediate lethal danger of getting shot before he could even get the gun pointed at his threat.

> Even when you have a gun, you may not be able to use it effectively to protect yourself.

Even if he had, he'd've been shooting into a car full of kids, only one of whom was posing an overt threat and he was positioned behind at least two others.

Training and Preparation:

WHEN YOU PLAN A NIGHT OUT WITH FRIENDS, HAVE A PLAN that allows you to maintain as much control as possible over your communication and transportation. Having a reliable cell phone is simply too easy and too inexpensive to not have one in this day in age. Keeping your vehicle with you or staying with those that you can count on to cooperate when you decide to leave is also important. If you are in an urban environment, having 'emergency' cab fare and the number of a reliable service or two is also a great preparation step.

> Firearms and alcohol do not mix. If you are going to drink, responsibly lock up your gun in a legal fashion.

Another thing that must be noted, based on my own experience: Even when it is a legal option for me to carry a firearm into a restaurant or bar, I generally choose not to when I am going out with friends, as I know that we will be consuming alcohol. I do not carry when I am drinking. And I rarely carry when I am around others who are. Life is full of compromises. If you want to carry a gun, I suggest avoiding bars and/or at least alcohol consumption.

How do I safely flee?

THERE IS NO "ONE" SAFE AND PERFECT WAY TO FLEE AN ARMED attacker. Let's face it, few of us can run as fast as we used to, and none of us can out-run a bullet traveling in excess of one-thousand feet per second. But if you choose to flee, here are a few things to consider:

Don't run in a straight line directly away from your attacker. As in Buddy's case, even a marginal marksman can get lucky at a short range, even if he's not given a lot of time to aim. Instead, force your attacker to make a good shot. This could mean running off at an angle, sometimes called a deflection shot, which is always a much tougher shot to make. You might also be able to run a short distance into darkness. Though not as good as actual cover, it still forces the gunman to fire blindly into the night. When available, it is best to move quickly, at an angle to real cover, such as a solid tree or the engine block of a car. The most dangerous places to be late at night are parking areas. Avoid them when you can. When you can't, scope them out for available cover should the need for it arise. Always create distance and angles while moving toward cover. That is your best chance to survive when someone is shooting at you.

When it comes to personal protection, an individual can do everything right and still be planted where they drop. Awareness is an important and useful tool, but self defense is an eclectic system comprised of many parts. You must use and master them all in harmony to enhance your chance of prevailing in a life or death struggle.

Chapter 5 - I'm Always Aware of My Surroundings

Mark Walters

WHAT HAPPENS WHEN YOU DO EVERYTHING RIGHT? Seriously. What happens when you are actually paying attention? What happens when your face is not buried in a phone, staring down like a blank slate as you walk back to your car at night? What happens when you are actually paying attention to your surroundings, awake, and aware? What happens when you are doing the right things? Think "it" can't happen to you?

Think again.

MR. LEE MICHAELS TOLD THE FOLLOWING STORY TO ME ON THE Armed American Radio show as I was broadcasting the program live from the 2010 Minnesota State Fair. He is the operations manager at my affiliate 1280 AM "The Patriot" in Minneapolis, Minnesota. The two of us struck up an instant rapport and a friendship that continues to this day. Lee's story is both harrowing and frightening-a life altering and extremely traumatic experience that will never be forgotten. It is an experience that will haunt and follow him for the remainder of his days on earth. Like most people I have come to know who have experienced this level of stress and trauma, Lee will never be able to shake the experience from his memory.

What makes events such as this even more frightening is that these are good people simply going about their daily lives, doing the things they enjoy doing, when in a horrible, terrifying instant they find themselves in fear for their lives at the hands of criminals. In an instant they find their fate being decided by monsters that don't care that they are attacking real people. These evildoers are not concerned with the fact that the woman they are violently forcing to the pavement may have just found out that she is pregnant. They have no concern whatsoever for the lifelong pain and suffering they are causing the child who witnesses a parent being beaten to within an inch of their life. They do not care that the elderly couple they are assaulting has just celebrated 60 years together. They simply do not care about their victims. They do not care about you and they certainly did not care about Lee.

Lee Michaels is a good man, a family man and a good friend to those who know him best. Like most good people, Lee is a valued employee and an esteemed member of his community, a great father, loving husband, and someone who spends most of his days working hard to support his family and be the best that he can be. He did not deserve what you are about to read.

IT WAS A TYPICAL NOVEMBER EVENING IN MINNESOTA, COOL and crisp, and Lee was on his way home from a "night of hockey" to the townhouse that he shared with his wife and children in the Minneapolis suburbs. As a radio station news and programming manager, he is no stranger to the bad things that happen to good people. Part of his job requires that he report this news and, as a result, he might be considered a little bit more aware of the realities of crime than the average Joe. As Lee put it to me when we talked, "I'm always aware of my surroundings." Lucky for him as it was his ability to remain aware that saved his life during a violent criminal ambush.

Coming home from a hockey game late in the evening sometime between 11 p.m. and midnight, Lee pulled into the parking lot of his townhouse complex as he had done countless other times. This time was a little different, as he remembered seeing someone on a bicycle. "I almost hit him," Lee told me as he recalled the evening. Stopping, he watched as the bike rider moved safely out of the way and out of his line of sight. Pulling into the garage, Lee maintained his situational awareness being "one of those people who usually leave the car running as the garage door closes," explaining that he does this just in case he needs "to get away or give up the car to save my life."

As the garage door closed, he finished his water bottle, tossing the empty container and grabbing some things from the car. He exited the garage through a side door and walked outside and stood in the front of his townhome. Looking up at his townhouse, admiring the fruits of his labor, he noticed the young man on the bike whom he had almost hit just moments earlier. He also noticed that something had changed. "This time he was walking towards me. I thought that was strange as I had just seen him on a bike, now he's walking towards me and then he asks me for some money," he said.

Lee responded to the man now up close to him on his own property, "No man, I just came home from a hockey game. I don't have any money for you. I wish I did." As he replied to the bicyclist, another man walked around the corner toward him carrying a firearm and as Lee put it, "This man was drawing down on me, so the first guy was a setup man. Right then, the first one moved around behind. He didn't have a mask on, but the one with the gun had a black hoodie and a skull-cap over his face and was asking me for money." Lee gave him a twenty-dollar bill, which was all the money he had on him at the time. Then the man asked him for his ATM card.

> The man I'd seen on a bike was now walking towards me, and this time he asked me for money.

Lee thought to himself, "Is this guy thinking I am going to give him my actual pin number?"

"You gotta give me more than that. I'm done with this, get on your knees," came the response from the masked, gun-wielding thug. "Get on your knees. I'm just gonna do him right here, I'm gonna fucking do him right now," the crazed punk with the gun told his partner.

The sickening reality of what was unfolding began sinking in. Lee began thinking about his family and about what was truly happening to him at that exact moment. He tried to grasp the fact that what was unfolding, as surreal as it seemed, was actually very, very, real. "I thought my wife was going to

38

come out and find me lying face down on the sidewalk right here, dead," he said.

Just then, at that exact moment, the gun-wielding criminal pistol-whipped him violently with the gun, striking him in the head several times. Being pistol-whipped and in fear for his life, with vicious blows raining down on the back of his head and neck, something remarkable happened.

He was able to keep his composure. His mindset changed. At that very instant Lee realized that he might very well be killed, murdered violently in cold blood in his own driveway mere steps away from the safety and security of his own living room and his family – all for nothing more than a lousy, crummy, $20 dollar bill – and he wasn't about to let that happen. He had made the decision to survive this encounter right there on the spot. He decided to live through this, no matter what. "I felt that everything was going to be all right and that I was going to get out of this. So I'm looking at the guy, I didn't want to look at his face too closely. I was looking at his boots, his clothing, when he told me I was going to take him to my bank."

> He was being severely beaten on the back of his head and neck. Then something remarkable happened.

The odds of survival drop significantly for anyone who actually gets into a vehicle with their assailant. Statistics show that the odds that a victim will be murdered rise sharply when a person is abducted against their will or willfully goes along in an attempt to satisfy their attacker. Lee Michaels decided that he was not going to allow this to happen to him. He would fight, and he would fight to win. As the situation continued to escalate, and as a gun-wielding madman was forcing him back into his garage, his determination and will to survive grew by the second. The gunman forced Lee to stand up, marching him into the garage with the gun at the base of his neck. As Lee got into the driver's seat of the car, the gunman's accomplice – who didn't have a gun – tried to get into the back seat of the car. The man would have to climb over Lee's daughter's car seat on the passenger side to do so.

> The odds that a victim will be murdered rise sharply when a person is abducted against their will.

With thoughts of survival running through his mind at a feverish pace, Lee frantically tried to dial 911 in his pocket on his cell phone. It didn't work … he had just purchased gas on his way home, and the receipt in his pocket was now covering the phone keypad. Feeling desperate, he didn't want the two punks who were holding his life in their hands to know what he was doing, so he gave up the attempt for the time being. Lee maintained his composure, although his mind was racing. "I knew the man with the gun couldn't get in the car from the passenger side. It was a one-car garage and I had parked really tight against the passenger-side wall. That's exactly what he tried to do … he walked around the car and hit me in the head again with the gun, just for good measure."

Still desperate, in survival mode and suffering from a splitting headache, Lee was paying very close attention to his situation when the criminal punk with the gun made a mistake. He blinked. He gave Lee the opportunity to act. "He opened the door and had to back into the seat and turn away from me, which is what he did and now had his hand with the gun against the wall. When he did that, I started the car and rocketed out of the garage as all 300 horsepower kicked in. I knocked him down and the guy in the backseat is now kicking the door because it's locked."

As he continued to back the car out, Lee watched the man in the garage stagger to his feet when the thug in the back seat of the car attacked. "He broke the windshield washer thing, grabbed the steering wheel and forced the car to the side, then jumped out and took off." Looking back towards the garage, Lee watched as the gunman also escaped. Furious and filled with adrenaline, he quickly dialed 911. Within minutes law enforcement arrived on the scene with K-9 units. Using the highly trained animals, they tracked the backseat punk to a nearby house. During questioning and a subsequent trial, he never gave up the name of his accomplice. As a result, the man with the gun was never caught; however, the unarmed man in the back seat, the punk Lee had originally encountered riding a bike upon returning home to his neighborhood that night, was convicted and served 54 months (4.5 years) in a Minnesota "Big House."

Lee is now a proud and highly trained gun owner, having received much of his professional training at the Sealed Mindset training facility in suburban Minneapolis, under the instruction of retired U.S. Navy SEAL Larry Yatch. Lee and his family have since moved into a new home.

When it comes to personal protection, the gray stuff between your ears is just as important as what type of gun you carry or how you carry it. Self defense isn't solely about your firearm.

Chapter 6 - Situational Awareness

Rob Pincus

ALL THE AWARENESS IN THE WORLD DOESN'T HELP YOU when you get ambushed. Humans are not built to be *aware* of more than one thing at a time, much less to be able to *focus* on more than one thing at a time. The modern world is full of distractions which decrease our odds of being aware of any particular person or warning sign. Even if you are aware of your surroundings and pick up on a potential threat, just as Lee Michaels did, you can still be outsmarted by criminals that are intent on turning you into a victim and who practice creating opportunities to do so. Going through life thinking that you will see the enemy coming or not ever get caught off guard is no better than relying on luck to keep you safe.

The Problem

LEE ACTUALLY DID TAKE SEVERAL STEPS TO BE AWARE OF HIS surroundings and to keep safe. But, while he may have been aware of the fact that danger existed, he wasn't committed to his own responsibility to protect himself enough to get the training and have the tools that would help him. Many people in today's world fall into that same trap. Telling yourself that you know what the warning signs are and that you know how to be alert simply isn't enough. Even if you do everything "right", you may still need to be prepared to defend yourself or your family. As Lee learned, once you've identified a threat, you need a plan to respond to it. Luckily, Lee was able to take advantage of an opportunity given to him by the armed attacker to improvise an action that may very well have saved his life.

Change the Story

IF LEE HAD TAKEN THE TIME AND EFFORT TO ARM HIMSELF prior to the attack that night, things might have gone very differently. On the one hand, being aware that he was moving into an area with a stranger, late at night and knowing that he would be forced to use a gun (or Taser, or Knife, etc.) if he needed to defend himself might actually have kept him from standing outside his garage for any length of time. It might also have changed his response to the first criminal. One of the first things you have to accept when you start carrying a gun is that you now have a higher obligation to avoid conflict and de-escalate situations whenever possible.

> Things may have transpired much differently if Lee had been carrying a firearm for self defense.

If Lee had placed one hand on a gun concealed under his jacket, while moving quickly towards his townhome, he may never have been stopped. If he had been, and he quickly responded that he had a $20 bill he could give the guy, the gunman may never have come out of the shadows. Of course, if he had been confronted by the gunman, he would've needed a *much smaller* window of opportunity to bring a well carried defensive firearm into his defense than when he needed to use his car.

Carrying a gun is no guarantee of safety... but, it does tend to change the behavior of those who are responsibly armed as well as present many more options for personal defense in a worst-case scenario.

The Four Levels of Awareness

The NRA has four levels of awareness:

Unaware

Aware

Alert

Alarm.

They are described as follows:

- Unaware - Most people spend a great deal of their lives in this state. In this condition they are totally unaware of what is going on around them. This is the most dangerous state of mind, and should be avoided at all costs. (It is also called "Condition White" in Colonel Jeff Cooper's Color Code.)

- Aware - Anyone bent on surviving and flourishing in life should spend most of their waking moments in this level of awareness. In this state you are aware of your surroundings. You know who is in your sphere of influence, and you have a good idea on whether or not they present a threat to you. (This is similar to "Condition Yellow" in the Cooper Color Code.) Opponents of awareness sometimes assert that a prolonged amount of time in this state may cause paranoia or result in a decreased quality of happiness in life. To counter this, it's important to note that the aware state has nothing to do with emotions or quality of life. It is simply a habit of living by a code which states "I will always be aware of my surroundings." People who routinely practice situational awareness do so as a matter of habit, with little cognitive effort.

- Alert - In this stage, you have identified a specific potential threat. In other words, something is wrong; something doesn't feel right; it could be nothing more than a gut instinct. But always trust your instincts. At this point, go on high alert, search out specific danger and be ready for anything. (This level of awareness is similar to the Orange Alert stage in the Cooper Color Code.)

- Alarm - The potential threat you saw in the "Alert" stage has proven to be real and credible. You are in imminent danger of being attacked, and you must immediately prepare your mindset and take every legal, moral and physical step to protect yourself. This is where all hell breaks lose. You bite, kick, scratch, scream and do whatever is necessary to stop the threat. Once you reach this level of awareness, you will fight until the threat stops even if that means using deadly force. (This level of awareness is similar to the Red Alert stage in the Cooper Color Code.)

The couple suspected Don but felt they had no way of proving it. The calls were never more than a few seconds long but long enough to make the point that they were in fact being watched and watched very closely.

Chapter 7 - Caroline and Rick Foster

Mark Walters

The following chapter is based on actual events. Because the case remains officially unsolved, the names of the individuals and locations have been changed to protect identities at the request of all parties involved.

To me, the story of Caroline and Rick Foster conjured up visions of a modern day Romeo and Juliet. Lifelong friends since kindergarten, the two were like peas and carrots as Forrest Gump might say. Growing up together in the Pennsylvania countryside, their families were the best of friends. Many friends and family members knew they were meant to be together from the time they were small children. "We pretended we were married when we were in the second grade, for crying out loud. I guess it was obvious even then," Caroline recalled with a smile.

Living in a quiet, small Pennsylvania town not far from the Revolutionary War battlefields of Valley Forge, Caroline and Rick spent every day together as children. "We were never apart. I mean I truly can't recall doing anything without him. Our families vacationed together during school breaks so we were literally always together," Caroline said.

As time passed, first grade became second grade; elementary school became middle school and high school soon followed. "High school is where our relationship really began to flourish," Caroline said. "I mean we're the same age and had known each other since we can remember but those formative years of raging hormones seemed to bring us closer," she chuckled. I would say we were about 15 years old when we realized that we were soul mates, that nothing was going to keep us apart."

> At the young age of fifteen, Rick and Caroline realized they were soul mates and that nothing would keep them apart.

As their high school years came to a close, both Caroline and Rick's families had discussed their children's futures. Caroline had graduated near the top of her class making the college of her choice a very real option. Rick, on the other hand, leaned more towards a vocational career choice following in the footsteps of his father, a highly skilled master mechanic and successful auto shop owner in town.

For the first time in their lives it seemed the two would be separated. Deciding they could do both, Caroline attended a nearby college, less than 85 miles and only two hours away in York. Rick stayed home and went to work with his father, learning the craft that had been in his family for as long as he remembered. "The distance was actually a good thing. I mean I could see him for dinner because we're like only eighty some miles away. Less than two hours apart made it easy to spend every weekend together when he wasn't working. Even if he was, I went home and helped him in the shop," Caroline said as her eyes drifted back in time.

Home one weekend for a family birthday party, Rick "made his move," as she recalled. "He asked me to marry him. I still had one year left in school but the answer was an immediate 'yes'. From there our lives seemed to go back to normal. I graduated soon after, moved home, married Rick and after his dad passed away I gave up my job managing a local insurance office and went to work at the auto shop."

> Finally, Rick proposed and they were married. It seemed they were on the way to their own 'happily ever after'.

It seemed only natural that kids would follow and within a few years the family had grown from Caroline and Rick to include three children, all roughly two years apart. "Along with that came the schedule that only a mother can appreciate," she said. "Rick and I had agreed that I would stop working and save the cost of day care, which any parent will tell you is incredibly expensive. So for the next few years, I spent every day driving to and from schools, after school events and sports activities. That's when everything began to change."

Joining a local soccer league for the kids had become the family past time. Mom would shuffle the kids to and from games and Rick would attend when his work schedule as the business owner would permit. With only one income and the ongoing daily expenses of running the business, it was vital to keep the shop open and making money. "He was busy and made it to the fields when he could. I never gave him any heat. He was providing for his family and doing a great job at it without my help at the office. I had no idea our lives were going to be turned upside down."

> And then Don entered the scene, and their lives were radically changed forever.

Caroline had noticed *him* looking at her when she signed the kids up at the soccer fields that morning. "I thought I recognized him. In fact I was sure of it. We had gone to school together and although he never gave me a hard time because he knew I had been 'dating' Rick my entire life, he asked me out from time to time only to be rebuffed with a smile. I never thought anything about it. Rick got a kick out of it and that was it. Now he was introducing himself to me as my oldest son's soccer coach."

Don was a nice guy, married to a woman whom Rick and Caroline didn't know with two kids of his own, one on his team with Caroline's son and another younger one who didn't play. "He would smile from time to time at me while I sat in the stands and on occasion would approach me after the practice or a game. I remember thinking it was odd that I never saw his wife attend any of the team functions, games or anything like that," she recalled. "It was becoming obvious he liked me. I could see it in his eyes and hear it in the way he spoke to me ... kinda' testing the waters with what could be considered a flirt, but always having an out if my reaction didn't meet his expectations. I was uncomfortable."

The apparent flirting began innocently enough according to Caroline but soon escalated to begin making her nervous. Finally, after a few weeks, she mentioned it to Rick after the kids went to bed one night. "He knew Don was coaching the kids and even reminded me about his attempts to hit on me when we were in high school. He kinda' blew it off but I knew it was bothering him."

As happens in so many of these cases, the flirtation became more aggressive at the ball fields, even in front of the kids. Constantly finding a reason to get near her, Caroline noticed the coach always peeking at her under his sunglasses when he should have been paying attention to the field. On one occasion he even sent one of the kids over to invite her to the sidelines. "It got to the point my son was asking me about it and mentioned it to his dad," Caroline remarked. He had approached my car after games or practices and asked if I could go get pizza with he and his kids. He brought me flowers and left them on the windshield of my SUV. Even though I never saw him do it, I knew it was him."

> The flirting escalated, making Caroline feel more and more uncomfortable.

In one case, Rick showed up unexpectedly, saw the flowers and approached Don after the game. Politely asking him to stop the games of cat and mouse with his wife, Rick remained calm. Don denied leaving the flowers and said as far as the invitations were concerned that he was only trying to be friendly. "I saw him slap Rick a 'high-five' and smile at him as Rick walked back to the car." Again, with his even disposition, Rick seemed to take it in stride almost proud that he had "won the girl", the admiration being shown towards his wife being viewed as some kind of an award. She figured she would blow it off and it would go away as long as she didn't reciprocate in any way, as Rick didn't seem too concerned with the situation.

> Finally, Caroline threatened to tell the league managers if Don didn't leave her alone.

It didn't go away.

"It got worse. The 'friendly' invitations continued. In fact I now felt uncomfortable enough that I asked him again to stop, reminded him I was married and that Rick didn't think his friendliness was funny. I was incredibly uncomfortable talking to him about it but threatened to tell the league managers if he didn't leave me alone."

Predictably, the attraction seemed to grow stronger after Caroline had politely asked her admirer to cease his unwanted advances. "The house phone would ring from unknown telephone numbers and the auto shop started getting prank calls. Two of the mechanics in the shop also started getting phone calls at home telling them they needed to quit their jobs. It was becoming unnerving. I knew it was him but couldn't really prove it."

In fact it was becoming downright scary. During the season ending league party, Caroline and Rick attended the awards function for the kids followed by a team party hosted by the coach and his assistants at a local VFW hall. Other than a few stares from the coach, nothing out of the ordinary seemed to happen. "I was glad Rick was there, " Caroline said.

Months passed with no incidents, and life seemed to get back to normal. The Foster's had moved on with their lives getting busier as the kids moved into the next school year and summer. The following years' soccer program had begun and Don was nowhere in sight. "I remember dreading going to the field. He had made the previous season so uncomfortable, and I just flat out didn't want to deal with it again this year." Apparently she wouldn't have too. The kids took to the fields with new coaches and some fresh young faces.

Approximately one month later the calls began again, first at the house then at the shop. This time they were threatening and frightening. "The voice was clearly disguised. I don't know how he did it but he would leave messages at the shop in the middle of the night describing what I had worn earlier that day or in some cases what I still had on. He knew when I was doing things,

For two months Don went away, then mysterious and threatening phone calls began coming in.

where I was and in one case he knew what I had to eat while I was out doing some shopping the day before." Caroline recalled.

The couple suspected Don but felt they had no way of proving it at this point. The calls were never more than a few seconds long but *long enough* to make the point that they were in fact being watched and watched very closely.

"Rick had considered seeking Don out, finding him and making his point, but without a 'smoking gun', he didn't feel right, he didn't feel we could prove it was actually him making the calls and the threats," Caroline said.

> Two months later Don and Rick exchanged words at a local store. The details will forever be a mystery.

Approximately two months after the calls stopped for the second time, the family bumped into Don at a local home improvement store one Saturday afternoon. Caroline watched as her husband motioned for her and the kids to stay behind at the register as he approached the smitten coach. She watched intently at the seemingly innocuous conversation, far enough away so as not to be able to make out what was said.

"There was nothing that gave the impression either one was upset at the other, but I know Rick enough to know that if he had approached Don to talk that he would certainly get his point across," she said. Walking back towards his family, Rick asked everyone to hurry to the car, told her everything was okay and assured her that Don wouldn't bother her again. "I asked him what he said to him, he told me not to worry about it, and I left it at that," Caroline said.

For the rest of their natural lives, Caroline and her children as well as Rick's mother and siblings will never know what was said that afternoon. Rick never spoke of it again. Two days later, he would be found by one of his employees, brutally beaten to death in his auto shop, left to die by the murderer on the dirty garage floor. Local police, after a thorough investigation, determined he had been murdered with a blunt object, which was never found. Robbery, they said, appeared to be the motive.

Given details of the stalking by Caroline, Don was questioned repeatedly by detectives but never charged. Noting that the store was in fact robbed of cash and some of Rick's personal belongings were stolen, several detectives believe the robbery was a cover-up instigated by the stalker. Because no solid proof was obtainable, Don remains a free man.

> **Two days later, Caroline's husband was found dead in the garage.**

The case remains open and Rick's wife, children and extended family and friends painfully await justice.

stalking
[staw-king]
noun
1. the act or an instance of stalking, or harassing another in an aggressive, often threatening and illegal manner: Stalking is now a crime in many states.

Chapter 8 - Defending Against Stalkers

Rob Pincus

The Problem:

STALKING IS A HUGE PROBLEM IN OUR SOCIETY. THERE IS technically and legally defined, "Stalking" and there is also quite a bit more of "one person giving another unwanted attention." The frequency of the latter leads us to sometimes not respond as assertively as we should to the former. Certainly, people can dig up an example or two of legally defined stalking that involve female stalkers, but they are the dramatic exception to the rule … so, I'm going to reference the overwhelming majority of the problem, the one that played a role here: An obsessive attraction to a woman that leads a man to behave irrationally.

When a man expresses interest in dating, courting or having sex with a woman and the woman is not 100% clear about her position on the topic, it can lead to misunderstandings and possibly to actions that become inappropriate on the man's part. If a woman who is not interested sends a mixed (or outright fraudulent) message that leads the man to think that she might be, naturally he is probably going to continue asking. If a woman tries to be coy or "play hard to get" with a man, she contributes to this pattern of behavior as well. By not saying that she is interested at first, but rewarding continued attention with an eventual "yes", the pattern of "no doesn't mean no" becomes understandably established in that man's mind ... and other men probably notice too. When communication is not clear, it can be hard to determine when persistence becomes legally defined "stalking".

Because of the somewhat blurry line, many people don't act as assertively as they should to address truly deviant stalking before it escalates to violence. If our society was less tolerant of persistence in making unwanted advances towards women, it would be easier for us to take assertive action against someone acting inappropriately. It would also be much easier to distinguish, very early on, if someone were innocently interested in some type of relationship or actually obsessed with a person and possibly posing a danger.

Change the Story:

IF CAROLINE AND HER HUSBAND HAD GONE TO THE POLICE AND moved towards having a restraining order put in place against Don right away, he may have removed himself from their lives sooner. When a psychologically deviant person has sociopathic tendencies, they become very good at rationalizing other people's actions to suit their agenda/perspective. It is much more difficult to tell yourself that a woman really is interested in you (but she is just stopped by her husband or "playing hard to get") if you are contacted by the police. Similarly, if Caroline had gone to the soccer league and informed them that Don was a problem, he may have been removed from the coaching position altogether. Of course, neither of those actions would definitely have stopped Don, but it is hard to say that they wouldn't have made it more difficult for his demented mind to create a narrative where he actually had a chance of a relationship with Caroline. In regard to the actual attack, where Rick was beaten to death in his garage, we'll never know what other precautions he could have taken to protect himself.

Training and Preparation

WOMEN SHOULD START BEING MORE ASSERTIVE WITH THE MEN in their lives, not only ones who are making advances, but even ones that they are in a relationship with. If a woman foregoes the all-too-common "I'm sorry, but I'm busy this weekend," when she really means, "Actually, I am not interested in going on a date with you. Ever," then it would become much more clear, much sooner, when a man was going to push his agenda forward regardless of the woman's lack of interest. Of course, this doesn't mean that women have to be rude. It may be as simple as telling your boyfriend or husband exactly where you would like to go on your next night out, instead of responding with "I don't care, you decide," when asked. Remember, even if you are in a relationship, single men may be watching your behavior to gauge whether or not you are disinterested in your current man or if you can be easily lead or manipulated. Putting a strong demeanor and confident attitude forward will send a clear message to anyone barking up the wrong tree. In regard to dealing with potential threats in your environment, trust your instincts … if you have a gut feeling that something isn't right with someone, don't turn your back on them. Stay focused and be ready to defend yourself at all times.

Personal safety tips concerning online stalking

Here is some important information according to women's personal defense expert, Cathy Steinberg, author of *The Fabulous Girl's Guide to Being Fearless*.

"Many a monster can now copy and save your pictures from your social site, rather than stalking you, to take your picture in person. The Internet makes it so much easier for a pervert to pursue you and follow your every move. Think before you do anything careless. Carefully consider the information being shared with strangers. Use a nickname, but if you choose to use your real name, then protect yourself with your privacy settings. Properly set controls keep the unwanted creepers out of your site and your pictures protected. All social sites have them. Once your private picture is out there, it is virtually impossible to get it erased completely off the Internet. The Internet never forgets. If you practice thinking strategically long enough, it will become a habit."

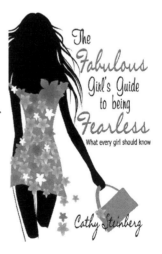

Bonus information from Rob Pincus

After reading this book, you may decide that you want to get yourself a defensive handgun and become part of Armed America. Personally, I would feel like we had done you a disservice if we didn't point you in the right direction. After decades of research and study of actual defensive use of firearms and working with thousands of students in hundreds of classes on scores of ranges across the United States and Europe, I have some very definite opinions on the topic of which type of handgun you should choose for personal defense. You know what I think about opinions? Some are worth more than others.

When you go to the gun shop, it is no different than going to the car dealership. You should do your homework beforehand and know what you want and why. Here is a chapter from one of my other books, *Counter Ambush*, that will get you started in the right direction!

Go to Appendix II at the end of this book for important training on picking the right defensive handgun for your personal protection needs.

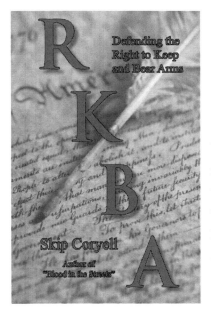

Columbine and Virginia Tech were not good omens. The victims there were unarmed sheep, who hid beneath desks and chairs, simply cowering as they died. They said "Baa" as they were being slaughtered. Something basic to our society has to change. It's time to stand and fight while we still can. And if our politicians tell us we can't protect our children in a daycare center, a post office, or a church, then we show them the door. We vote them out. We recall them. We take out the trash! That's the attitude that America was founded on. Somewhere along the timeline, America has lost it's way, we've lost our instinct for survival; it's no longer "fight or flight"; it's just plain "cower and die"!

Don't cower in the face of crime! Read this book and make your stand. That's one of the themes in Skip Coryell's new book *RKBA: Defending the Right to Keep and Bear Arms*.

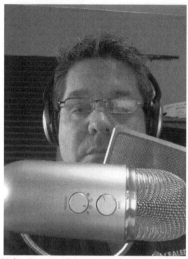

Author Mark Walters recording promo's and liner's for station affiliates at his home studio

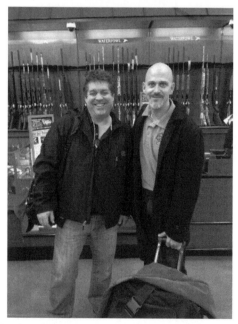

Authors Mark Walters and Rob Pincus departing a CCW Expo event at Gander Mountain in Houston TX

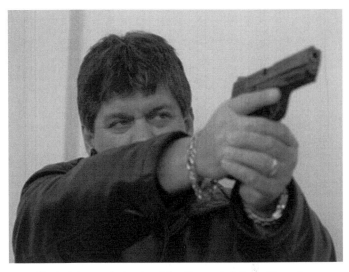

Mark doing a photo shoot for Concealed Carry Magazine
(Photo by Oleg Volk)

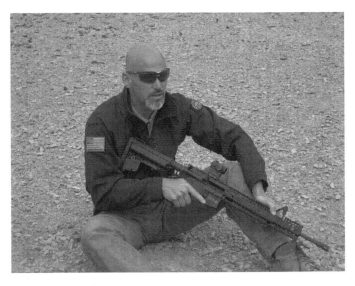

Although Rob is best known for teaching defensive pistol skills, he
also has developed a Combat Focus® Carbine course.

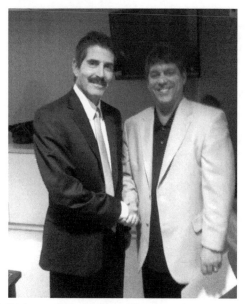

Mark Walters visits with host John Stossel in the Fox News Television studios in New York City after taping an episode of the Stossel Show, More Guns, Less Crime

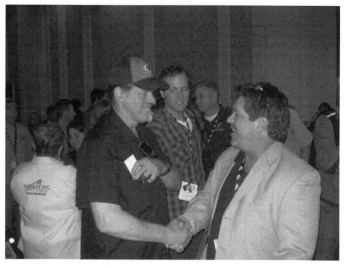

Mark Walters and Ted Nugent confer at SHOT Show in Las Vegas

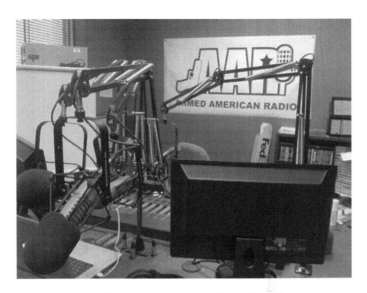

View from the guest seat in the AAR studio

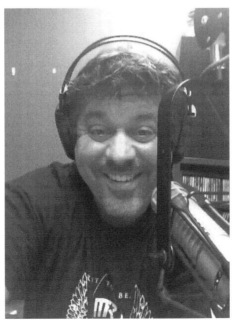

In the studio sporting a Madison Rising T-Shirt

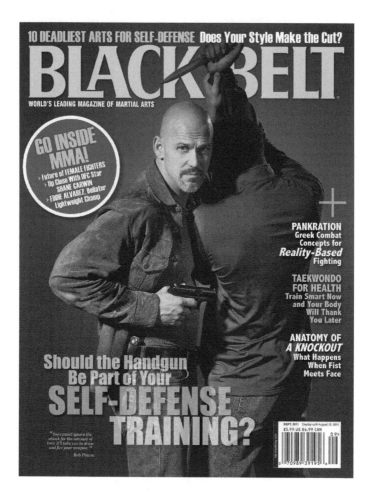

Rob Pincus was the first Instructor specializing in Defensive Handgun Use to be featured on the cover of the prestigious *Black Belt* Magazine.

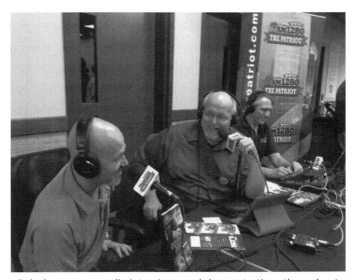

Rob does many media interviews and demonstrations throughout any given year to educate "non-gun" audiences about responsible armed defense.

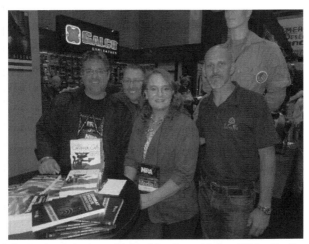

Rob at a booksigning with his friends and fellow White Feather Press authors, Kathy Jackson and Mark Walters

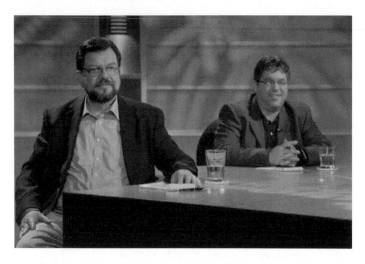

Mark and AAR regular contributor David Codrea on the TV set of
American Trigger Sports Network filming an episode

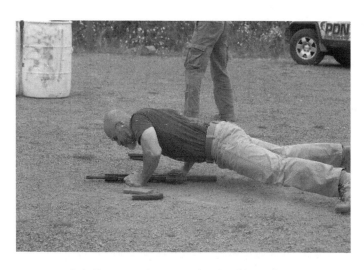

Rob Pincus on the range showing his students
how to work and train hard!

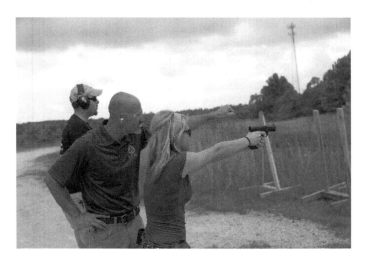

Rob giving a pointer to his daughter during a Combat Focus®
Shooting course in 2012.

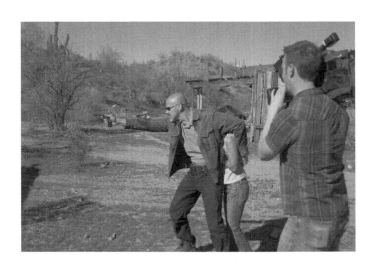

The great Rob Pincus in action showing how to
protect and defend the ones you love

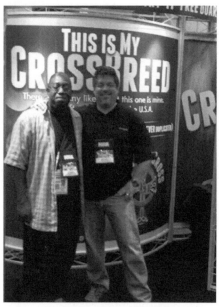

Mark Walters and AAR producer Sean "Seanto" Young together at a book signing event with Crossbreed Holsters at 2013 NRA annual convention in Houston

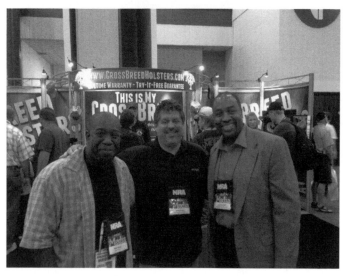

Mark Walters with Sean Young and Black Man with a Gun, Rev, Kenn Blanchard at 2013 NRA convention

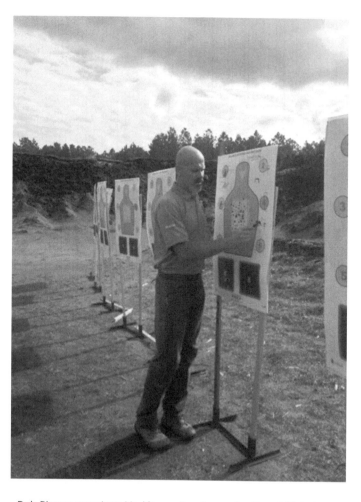

Rob Pincus examines Mark's results after a shooting drill during a
Combat Focus® Shooting class

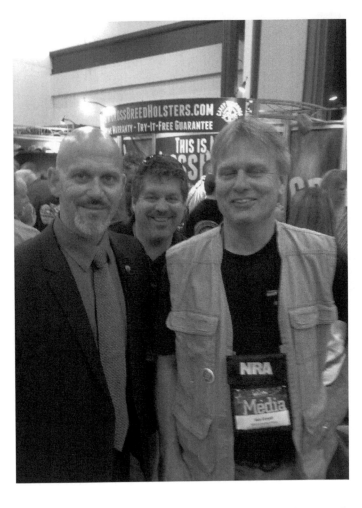

Mark sneaks into a photo of Rob Pincus and publisher Skip Coryell

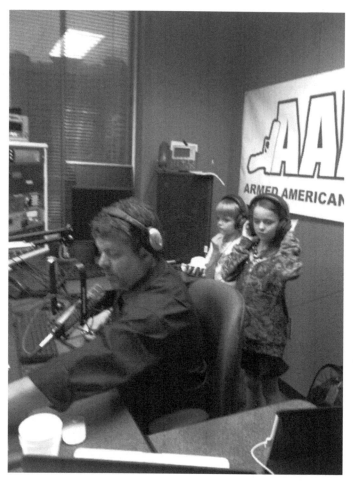

Marks children enjoy watching dad bring AAR to the nation during a live broadcast

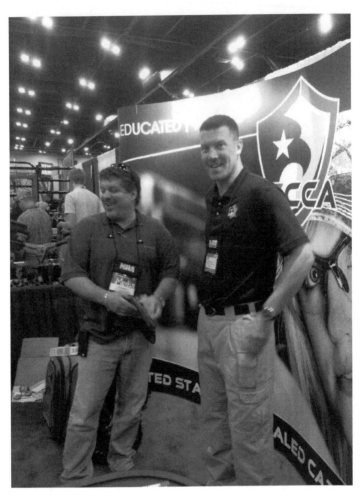

Mark Walters and USCCA founder Tim Schmidt at the USCCA booth during the 2013 NRA annual convention

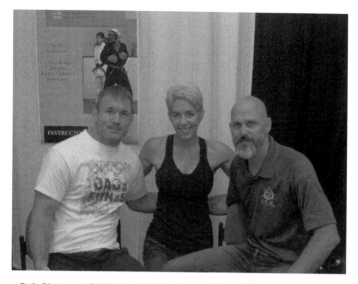

Rob Pincus at 2012 Martial Arts Super Show with Kelly Muir, 2012 BlackBelt Magazine Woman of the year, and Matt Hughes, Former UFC Champion

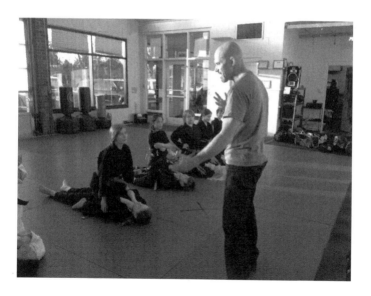

Rob Pincus enjoys teaching young people the art of self defense

In August 2002, on a Wednesday evening approaching midnight, John K. walked out of his front door on a business trip to Charlotte, North Carolina. He had no idea that his destiny included a rendezvous with evil.

Chapter 9 - The "Not So Restful" Stop

Mark Walters

THE TRANSPORTATION INDUSTRY, NAMELY THE HEAVY HAUL segment of the long-haul trucking industry, employs millions of Americans. It is a tough, gritty and highly competitive business. Although most of us think of the truck driver when we think about the trucking business in general, the driver himself (or herself) is actually just one of many components that keep the nation's wheels of commerce spinning. John K. is an example of the other side of the trucking business. He represents the side of a cutthroat industry that most of us rarely see: he is the sales executive responsible for putting the nation's economy – everything from raw materials to finished goods – on board the truck to its final destination. A common saying within the freight industry is, "If you can see it, it's been on a truck." The job requires significant travel to and from company-owned freight terminals, as well as meeting customers at their own places of business across the country. Tonight John was heading to one of his company facilities.

Like many of the people I have interviewed over the years, John is a long-time friend and this story is a personal one, as we have known each other for many years. He is proof that most of us know someone who has been a victim of some type of criminal activity. I was shocked when I found out about his harrowing ordeal, but again not *surprised* that it had happened. John will be the first one to tell you how thankful he is to be alive today, because he realizes that the outcome could have turned out much, much worse than it did. He is also never going to forget the terrible ordeal he suffered that fateful early morning. He tries to keep it out of his mind, while at the same time using it as a reminder to remain vigilant at all times.

John is a quiet, disciplined man, a great manager, and a fantastic "people" person. I'm convinced that it is his very good-natured personality that allowed him to survive his frightening, face-to-face brush with malevolence to make it home alive and uninjured afterward. Like all potentially life-threatening encounters with evil, John's story is compelling, eye opening, and one that should be heard by everyone who lives their own life thinking that it can't happen to them.

Here's how it happened to one good man, early in the midnight morning hours at a lonely, desolate South Carolina rest stop.

Leaving his wife and kids routinely for business meetings on a fairly regular basis, John was no stranger to nights away from home. This trip promised to be no different. "It was a normal trip to our dedicated fleet operation in Charlotte," John told me later. "Sometimes I would leave late to observe the crews on night shift, so leaving home between 11 and midnight for the ride to Charlotte was not out of the ordinary for me."

This night held something different in store for him though, something that he had no way of knowing would occur, something that left him totally unprepared for its swiftness, its intensity and its violence. "I was never a gun owner," John said. "I had fired them over the years, and certainly had no fear of them, but there just wasn't a part of me that made me feel like I needed a weapon." Pulling out of his driveway late that night and into the midnight darkness, John thought about the drive and the work ahead of him as he headed toward Charlotte from his home in suburban northern Atlanta. Approximately two hours into the drive, the time came for a rest stop break from the monotonous quiet loneliness of the interstate highway late at night. Some time between 1:30 and 2:30 in the morning, feeling a little restless, John pulled off of Interstate 85 and into the Hartwell, South Carolina rest area for a much-needed break just inside the South Carolina border.

"It was a quiet and actually very peaceful drive. I tend to get a lot of thinking done when I drive, especially late at night. I don't mind the road at night and in fact it almost relaxes me. I like driving at night," John said. Pulling into the rest stop, he fumbled for some change to get something cold to drink from one of the machines after he would finish visiting the restroom.

"I remember there not being anyone around me, and it was just like many other times I drove this route. Stop, head to the restroom, get a drink and finish the remainder of the drive," he said.

"I exited my car and headed toward the restroom around the corner on the side of the building when I noticed a young woman on a pay phone in between the men's room and the ladies' room. She didn't seem out of place at the time," John said. Walking past the young woman on the phone, John entered the bathroom. "It was empty. I looked around and there was no one else in the place. It was very quiet."

Finished using the bathroom, John had turned toward the sink when his night took a turn for the worse. In fact, what he saw would alter the remainder of his life and forever change the way he thought about his own safety, the safety of his family, and the responsibility to be ready to defend his own life at a moment's notice.

As he finished using the restroom, he turned around to find two young, white men standing directly in front of him. "I never heard them come in. The first was about five feet, eight inches tall and pointing a handgun directly at my face, his arm outstretched. He was about five feet away from me, I would guess. Blocking the door was another guy about six feet, three inches tall. He was holding what looked like a table leg of some sort that had been whittled down to almost look like a small bat. He scared me more than the guy with the gun," John recalled.

With a loaded handgun pointed directly at his face, and a thug with a table leg blocking the only exit from the restroom, John was trapped. "Mister, we're desperate. We want your cash now. We don't want to hurt you but we're desperate," said the robber holding the gun.

Reaching behind him, heart racing and saying nothing, John reached into his back pocket and retrieved his wallet. "I don't know if I should say it this way, but I was lucky in that I had stopped at an ATM earlier in the day and grabbed a couple of hundred dollars in cash for the trip. Strange because I don't normally carry much cash on me," he said. He extended his arm, his wallet in his hand. The man with the pistol pointed directly at him said, "We don't want your wallet, mister. Not your credit cards or anything else. Just hand me the money you have in your pocket. Take it out and give it to me now, and we won't hurt you." John continued, "I was going to take my wallet and toss it to him when he said that, so I stopped and did what he said. The guy with the table leg was making me very nervous. I remember thinking that I didn't want that gun to go off, but for some reason, the man with the club was even scarier. He made me very, very nervous."

After taking the money from John's wallet, the thug with the gun ordered John into the stall. "You go in there and you stay for 15 minutes. Don't you even think of coming out for at least 15 minutes." Keeping his eye on both men, John did as ordered at gunpoint and went into the stall nearest him, closing the door behind him. "I had already made the decision that if I had been ordered face down or told to kneel and face away from them that I was going to fight. I was ready mentally for that. I was not going to comply with an order like that. I knew what that would mean, and I was ready to fight for my life at that point."

Now in the stall for approximately 10 minutes, and frightened at what lay outside, John opened the door and cautiously exited the restroom. Thankfully there was no one in the area. "It was obvious to me then that the girl on the payphone was an accomplice acting as a lookout. It all made sense in hindsight," John told me.

Scared and wanting out of there, John made for his vehicle and headed out of the rest stop. Traumatized and in shock and not really thinking clearly, he made it up the freeway a bit before thinking to himself that he had to report the incident to the police. Once he was safely out of the rest area and down the road, he dialed 911 and reported the armed robbery. Dispatchers immediately turned his call over to the South Carolina Highway Patrol, when the dispatcher on the phone told him that "no one was in the area to stop to take his statements" and there was nothing they could do about it.

With no description of any vehicle and no help from highway law enforcement, it became painfully apparent to him that he was plain old out of luck. "They told me they would make a report of the incident and report it as a statistic at that rest stop and alert other officers that the robbery had occurred, but other than that, nothing. It was very surreal. I kept on going and continued on my trip. Went to work like nothing happened and tried to put it out of my mind," he said.

John is a man of high personal integrity and values. I sat spellbound by his statements throughout our conversation, and thought about my own many trips over the years on similar stretches of freeway at the same time of night. This could easily have been me, I thought to myself. This could be my mother and father as they head back to Florida on their bi-annual runs, or any number of friends or family members. This *does* happen to people we know, not just those we read about in newspapers and online reports or sensational television news stories read by news anchors as if it were some kind of fictional show. This is *real*. My heart felt for him as I watched his eyes shift, envisioning in his own mind's eye the events of that night.

"In hindsight, which is always 20/20, if I had been armed I would have waited until I was ordered into the restroom stall before having an opportunity to draw my weapon on an already drawn gun pointed at my face. If it came down to them ordering me to the floor or to lie down, I would have had no choice but to draw and fight," he told me. "Unfortunately, I didn't have a weapon of my own, but then fortunately, I was unhurt. Imagine two armed criminals actually keeping their promise not to hurt me. I'm very lucky."

Since that frightening incident in the Hartwell, South Carolina rest stop early in the morning of a balmy August night in 2002, John has obtained his Georgia carry permit. Like so many other common, ordinary people I have had the opportunity to write about over the years, John vows never to be caught off guard again. Thankfully he is alive to make that promise to himself and his family. He is now a gun owner and continues an exemplary career as one of the most well-respected corporate officers of a major trucking concern in North America.

No one can <u>always</u> be around other people, nor would they want to be, but isolation is a problem for people wishing to avoid becoming a victim of crime. Criminals don't like witnesses; they don't like being interrupted while they work.

Chapter 10 - The Problem: Isolation

Rob Pincus

ISOLATION IS A HUGE TOOL OF THE PREDATOR. BAD GUYS SEEK to isolate you from witnesses and potential aid. There are very few incidents of "out in the open" crime happening in crowded places. And when crimes do occur in public spaces, such as banks, the bad guy almost always seeks to remain inconspicuous, using notes and subtle threats, instead of overt confrontation. Knowing this, simply doing the best you can to avoid isolation is a great way to increase your personal safety and to avoid being targeted as a victim.

While the meaning of "isolation" may at first glance mean that you never want to be alone, remember that you really need to avoid being isolated *with* a potential threat. After all, if you were truly alone, there wouldn't be a bad guy there to threaten you. Remember that in John's story, he did see a woman on the phone. Now, personally, seeing a woman on the phone at a rest stop at 2:00 am is something that would throw up a bit of a red-flag for me. I'm not say-

> To increase your personal safety, always do your best to avoid isolated areas.

ing that I wouldn't have gotten out of the vehicle or used the restroom, but it would certainly have aroused my suspicion that something wasn't right with the world, even if it was just a problem that she was having with her vehicle.

Change the Story:

WHAT IF JOHN K. HAD NEVER STOPPED? WHILE IT MAY SEEM overly simplistic, it is a very real option. Trying to find ways in our everyday routines to avoid potential isolation is an easy way to be safer. If John had brought a beverage with him, or planned his stops around populated areas with all night convenience stores or truck stops, he could've avoided the isolation of the interstate rest-stop.

> Learn to think out of the box, trying creative, unusual ways to enhance your own personal safety. He could have simply locked the door.

What if John K. Had locked the bathroom door? While it may seem unusual, the fact is that the bathrooms were a point of isolation where John was going to be *pre-occupied* and could easily be trapped. Thinking ahead, if John K. had turned the lock on the door behind him, taken care of his business and then unlocked the door and left, the worst thing that might have happened would have been a slightly, inconvenienced fellow traveler. Locking the door to a "public" space for your own protection in the middle of the night may be outside the social norm, but it is a simple step that can keep you safe and be easily explained if you were to be confronted by an employee. Even if a police officer or security guard happened to stop by in the few minutes that the door was locked, a simple explanation is probably all that would be needed. Ultimately, if you are not doing anything nefarious on the other side of the locked door, there isn't much that anyone could say or do about it after the fact, as you apologized for any potential problem you may have caused and headed on down the highway.

Preparation and Training:

WHENEVER YOU ARE GOING TO BE TRAVELING, YOU SHOULD take a few minutes to think about your route and your scheduled stops. For times when you don't plan or when there are unanticipated needs to stop, you should give yourself a set of guidelines about when and where it makes sense to take non-emergency detours on your trip. Populated areas obviously make the best choices. Simply waiting until you see another car exit to use a rest stop or slowing down and looking ahead to see how many cars are in a rest area already can be simple ways to avoid isolation as well.

> Plan your late-night stops at populated areas. This is the safest and best choice.

Thinking about how you can quickly and surreptitiously secure a room or space in a public area is another way that you can plan ahead to avoid being trapped by a predator. You can even carry a simple rubber door stop in your jacket or purse that can be used to at least slow down or deter a would-be attacker trying to follow you into a restroom or other public access space.

Evil people, not inanimate objects, commit evil deeds ... guns in the right hands, the hands of law-abiding people, do good things.

Chapter 11 - We Can Triumph Over Evil

Mark Walters

The Incredible Life Journey of Mr. Tony Walker

NO OTHER TRUE CRIME TALE OF TERROR I'VE WRITTEN OR read about to date has saddened me more than *Because I Needed the Money* as told to me by Mr. Jorrick Landry, which appeared in our first book, *Lessons from Armed America,* under the chapter of the same name. Forced to defend his family with a gun while being terrorized by evil, Jorrick Landry killed his family's attacker. In the process, a stray bullet from his own gun also killed his 10-year-old son, who was sitting in the back of the family SUV, directly behind the scene of unfolding violence. The horrors I was told, and the devastation to the Landry family that ensued, are memories that I will never be able to put out of my head. I can't even begin to imagine what the family endured, or how they have coped over the years with the tragedy that befell them through absolutely no fault of their own other than being at a location that would find them face to face with evil at a time of evil's choosing. Without a doubt, it had the most impact on me as a writer, as a father, and as a human being that no other incident has been able to match.

This one comes close.

Never did it occur to me that I would someday hear another tale so devastating as to put it on a scale with the tragedy endured by the Landrys. When hearing of these events from the mouths of those who lived through them, I am always struck by the candid frankness of the victims. Their willingness to recount the terror they experienced is almost therapeutic. It seems almost as if they have an inner desire to help others, to see that the events that forever changed or ruined their lives are never experienced by another. I have also found that the glue that holds these incredible people together after such a horrifying, life-altering tragedy is their faith. Faith in God, be it newfound or a strength that existed before their encounter with evil, seems to always overcome the wreckage forced upon them.

I have also found that there is a lesson to be learned, and we need to be thankful to those who are willing to recount such personal devastation for the benefit of others. I have watched news reports of terrible tragedy happening to otherwise normal people, and I have often wondered how they cope. The loss of a child is a loss that no parent should ever have to endure, whether it comes through accidental violence, natural occurrence, or crimes so vile that they defy our logic and ability as humans to even comprehend the dissoluteness of those who can perpetrate such an act on a fellow human being. It is a stark reminder that terrible things happen to good people, yet *good can come from anything,* if only we let ourselves see through the evil and refuse to let it prevail.

94

That describes no one better than Mr. Tony Walker. Tony Walker is the quintessential example of good prevailing over evil. His life story is one born of such an act of criminal terror that most of us are unable to comprehend. His incredible journey from a witness to unconscionable violence as a little boy – just 10 years old – into a man of incredible integrity will leave you awestruck. He reminds us all that we can *win in* the face of utter horror.

I met Tony when I ran a contest on the Armed American Radio broadcast. The contest consisted of an AAR sponsor of the national radio show giving away products to a lucky participant or participants whose name I announced live on the air during the Armed American Radio show. One of the winners was a man named Tony Walker, selected at random by my producer during the live program. I announced his name on the air and a few days later, I received the following email:

"Dear Mr. Walters,

I've wanted to get in touch with you and tell you how your book (Lessons from Armed America) helped me deal with my mother's murder, but didn't want to bother you. But, since I won the AAR Giveaway what better opportunity! I work on 3rd shift Sunday nights so I did not hear the show live. I download the podcast and listen usually on Tuesday afternoons. About 2 a.m. I was checking my Twitter feed and I saw the tweet from you that said my name and I screamed. Someone at work said, 'What is it?' and I said, 'I GOT IT! I GOT IT!' I wish you could have seen the scene!

"Just so happens, I bought and read your book you co-au-

thored about 3 weeks ago. I am sure that it has helped a lot of people, but I read it from a perspective that most people haven't. And I can honestly say that it helped me deal with some things. It's hard to put into words, but as I read it, it took me back almost 20 years ago just like it was yesterday.

"I am 28 years old now. In 1994 my step dad (my real dad is unknown) murdered my mother, when I was a 10-year-old boy. I was in my room playing with a neighbor when my step dad came in the front door. I recall hearing my mother say, 'Don't do it!' but I never heard the gunshot. (Your book was the first time I have heard the words 'auditory exclusion.' I'm not sure how one would explain the non-shooter experiencing auditory exclusion, but it happened even though neighbors heard the shot go off from their homes.)

"Even though I didn't hear the shot, I 'knew' something happened. (God/intuition?) I immediately ran through the house and right there it seemed like time sped up and slowed down all at once. I saw my mother lying on the floor. I still remember how she was lying against the wall. I didn't stop to look. I kept running until I exited the house and ran to a neighbor's house. But that scene will never leave me I guess. When I exited the house he reached for me with his bloody hands and I ran away. Before I went to bed that night (my baby sitters became my parents that night and still are today), I took a bath and I remember washing my mother's blood off of my arm. Tough for anyone, much less a 10-year-old boy.

"After the events transpired and we went to trial I learned

everything. He put a .22 in her mouth and tried to shoot her but the gun jammed. It left a circular cut on her lip, which I had to look at a picture of and say that that wasn't there earlier in the day. After the gun jammed she ran out the kitchen to the laundry room. In the laundry room he pulled out a .40 pistol and shot her in the head. The bullet entered the bridge of her nose, exited out of the back of her head, went through a window, and hit the side of my neighbor's house. They said she died immediately. After a couple of hours they took him to jail and they told me in the driveway that my mother was dead. That was March 22, 1994, three days before my mother's birthday.

"After witnessing my mother suffer beatings, stalking, threats, and ultimately being shot, I didn't swing to either extreme. I am not anti-gun in one ditch. I also am not in the other ditch repeating the violence I grew up with. I got my CWP in 2006. This month on March 24, my wife will take her CWP class.

"I consider myself blessed that I was adopted by people who love me, grew up in a home that was stable, became a Christian, and gave my life to serve the Lord. I have a wife, a 2-year-old daughter, and 5-month-old twin boys and it is my job to protect them. I love them. I grew up in a home with a step dad of hate and guns used to promote fear. I want my family to grow up with a dad of love and see guns used to know that I will protect them because I love them.

I have wondered what I am supposed to be doing with my life. Evangelism, missionary, church planter, pastor have all crossed my mind. I used to think I knew; now I am not sure. I do know, however, that the Lord has protected me, and a life that could be bitter and hateful is one that is trying to serve Him. I am just not sure in what capacity yet. I have had a small radio program since 2004 that airs weekly here in Anderson, SC, The Bible Broadcast. I also have my life story and radio archive on my website, www. preachertony.com.

"It seems lately though I have been thinking a lot, a whole lot, on what happened that day almost 20 years ago and how I can use it to help other people (and make sure it never happens to me or my family also).

"Sorry to write such a long letter! I'm glad that my name was picked for the prize and I hope that my story has been a blessing to you. If nothing else you can tell people that just because someone grows up around violence doesn't mean they will turn out that way, and you know someone to prove it.

Thanks so much!

Tony Walker"

I know. I can hear what you're thinking. Like you, I sat and tried to place myself in Tony's shoes. How on God's earth would I handle something so horrible? Where do people who experience such pain and tragedy gather their strength? How do they go on? It is almost impossible to comprehend surviving such tragedy unscathed, and I can only hope that God would give me the strength that Tony has found.

Tony and I exchanged emails and he brought his life story to Armed American Radio on the 3-18-2012 broadcast. He agrees with me that whenever we hear of a tragedy when a gun is used to murder, rape, rob a good person, the media always blame the gun and not the criminal who chose to misuse the gun to commit his or her evil deed. I was fascinated with his response to witnessing this horrible event that changed so many lives around him and thought it incredibly important to bring his message, with his blessing, to as many people as we can reach. His message is that we cannot blame an object for the death of his mother, but rather blame must be placed where it belongs, on the person who chooses to use the tool for evil deeds.

Too many times, the media, gun-grabbing groups such as the Brady Campaign, the Violence Policy Center, and too many politicians to count, demonize us as gun owners. Tony's message of responsibility is a powerful one. Evil people, not inanimate objects, commit evil deeds. He told me that he couldn't place the blame for his mother's murder on Mr. Glock or the piece of polymer and steel that he invented. No, Tony understands that bad people do bad things … that things by themselves can be neither good nor bad, but it is people who choose to commit evil deeds.

Tony Walker now spreads the message that guns in the right hands, the hands of law-abiding people, do good things. He believes this is a message that needs repeating every day to those who would choose to demonize gun owners or the object itself, rather than focus their attentions on the criminal.

Since I received his original email, Tony has joined me on air to discuss his life story to a national radio audience. In discussing this chapter of the book with him via email, I have come to believe that there are simply some people who are given to us by God as examples of how we should live our lives. Tony is one of those people to be held up as an example of what can come from evil when we refuse to let it win. This excerpt from another email he sent me regarding this chapter appearing here in *Lessons from Unarmed America* is further evidence of Tony's true goodness as a man:

> *"I am truly honored, Mark. As awful as the events are, I am thankful that I have had an opportunity to help others. Thank you so much for making that door of opportunity much larger than it would be had our paths not crossed. When I read your book, little did I know that my story would be able to help others in a future edition of it. From the bottom of my heart, thank you. Together with my story and your national influence and name I hope that we can help as many people as possible."*

As I did during the writing of the Landry story several years ago, I have done much soul-searching after reading, writing about, and interviewing Tony Walker. As much as I would like to believe that I could move forward with my life if I had experienced an event like this, I am not yet convinced that I would be capable. We have all seen the terrible stories on the news of the parents who lose their children in accidents, to criminals, fires, and other unimaginable tragedy. I am reminded of the mother who lost both of her parents and all of her children in a house fire in southern Connecticut. I have seen her interviewed, and to this day I do not know where her strength comes from. I am not afraid to admit that I may not be strong enough to go forward. Some of the horrible acts of evil we read about and see every day are so terrible that you wonder why the survivors would even *want* to go forward.

Tony and his family reside in South Carolina. He has dedicated and given his life to God. Together he and his wife are raising a beautiful family including twin sons.

Unbelievably, his stepfather was given a 30-year sentence and will be eligible for parole in 2014.

It is a well-established fact that many acts of violence, especially those against women, are committed by hands that were at one time known and trusted by the victim.

Chapter 12 - Domestic Violence

Rob Pincus

WHILE IT WOULD BE LUDICROUS TO SUGGEST THAT TONY Walker wasn't a *victim* of violence (he lost his mother and who knows how much of his childhood to a horrific act of violence), his mother was the one who was murdered in this story, so I am going to focus on her. Domestic violence is one of the most insidious problems in our society. Often, lower levels of domestic violence, including stalking, are precursors to murder. It is a well-established fact that many acts of violence, especially those against women, are committed by hands that were at one time known and trusted by the victim. Tony's mother, killed by his step-father, was apparently a victim of domestic violence ("*…After witnessing my mother suffer beatings, stalking, threats…*") before she was a victim of murder.

The Problem:

TOO OFTEN IN OUR SOCIETY, CRIMES ARE NOT REPORTED. Whether it is fear of the attacker, fear of society's judgment, fear of being labeled a "victim" or simply fear of the hassle of reporting a crime and dealing with a sometimes-less-than-awesome legal system, *fear* is the most common reason for people not reporting crimes.

People who commit crimes demonstrate a disregard for the social contract, a lack of discipline and a lack of concern for the welfare of others. Without outside influence it is illogical to assume that their behavior will stop. In fact, it has been shown that without outside interference, especially in the case of domestic abuse and many cases of stalking, the problem only gets worse. Victims need to take action. Whether that action is active self-defense, reporting the crime to the authorities or other protective measures (relocating, seeking private-protective services, asking a third party to intervene on your behalf, etc.) or any other measure doesn't specifically matter. Victims (and witnesses!) of crimes need to be encouraged to take action. This starts with our children, who shouldn't be taught to "turn the other check" or "just ignore" the bullies they encounter in grade school. It continues with our teens and young adults who should be taught to think critically and not blindly rely on others. This carries on into our adult years when we should do more than just *hope* a bad situation we are in will get better.

> Too many crimes go unreported. The victims are afraid, but, most often, their best method of self defense is to TAKE ACTION!

Change the Story:

IF TONY'S MOTHER HAD GOTTEN THE POLICE INVOLVED, HER husband might have changed his behavior. He might have been deterred from further violence. He might have been arrested and charged with crimes that resulted in jail time and a break in the hostility that was apparently taking place in the household that would've allowed Tony's mother to distance herself from him. She might have gotten a restraining order that would've caused her husband, out of fear of further ramifications from his deviant behavior, to change his way of life or, at least, move on to another target. At this point, many people often think that the act of going to the police, or talking to anyone, about the problems might have 'provoked' further violence. Before you let that thought go too far, remind yourself that Tony's mother was ultimately *murdered*! There was no escalation possible.

> In domestic violence scenarios, the trust and hope factors often prevent the victim from taking decisive action.

I believe that the only change in behavior that will be caused by a victim taking action in this situation is one of two possibilities: The bad guy takes action that he would've eventually taken anyway (but, at least the victim, the police and anyone else alerted to the problem can be more "on guard") or, the bad guy backs down in the face of someone who clearly is going to resist victimization. In these situations, it is often a stretch to suggest that better personal defense training or preparation would've helped Tony's mother. Because of my work in law enforcement, teaching of Women's Assault Prevention courses and my work as a consultant to the Wrong Woman™ Program, I have spent a great deal of time researching domestic violence and sexual assault. Because of the trust and hope factors that play such a strong role in guiding the victim's behavior, it is highly unlikely that physical training, skills or equipment would have been likely to change the outcome. All the training in the world and the best equipment available is meaningless if the person with them refuses to accept the reality of their threat or does not possess the will to take action.

Preparation and Training:

Gen. Gordon R. Sullivan, Chief of Staff of the US Army from 1993-1995, wrote a book titled *Hope is Not a Method.* I have used that phrase many times over the last twenty years to help people understand that they need to be proactive. Hope, trust and faith might get you by on a rainy day, but they alone are not enough to weather a true storm. Preparing your self mentally to take action, to refuse to be a victim, to hold others accountable for their transgressions and to recruit the help of others is the best way to prepare for the emotional and social trauma that comes with taking action. The existence of a con-

> Hope is not an effective defense against domestic violence. Prepare yourself mentally and refuse to be a victim!

flict is defined by the existence of an aftermath. Often, the aftermath of our personal defense conflicts have less to do with physical issues than they do mental. Overwhelmingly, I have seen people deal much better with the aftermath issues from conflict when they have done *something* in their own interest or to stop the actions of their threat. When the opportunity presents itself, take action against evil.

Alone, aware of her surroundings and looking for any possible dangers, she noticed a blue Dodge truck and a sedan parked across from her own vehicle but it's what she didn't see next that would alter the rest of her life.

Chapter 13 - The Amanda Collins Story

Mark Walters

IT IS NEVER EASY ASKING ANOTHER HUMAN BEING TO RELIVE what is, without fail, the most frightening, painful and horrible experience of their lifetime, and although I am able to transfer the words that I hear to paper, I am never able to convey the sound of the sheer emotion on the other end of the phone, the distance in the eyes or the sadness and terror I see on the face from across the desk. Trust me, it never gets any easier. In fact, just when I think I have heard the absolute worst of the worse, the ultimate story of human degeneracy and depravity against a fellow human being, another one comes along.

What happened to Amanda Collins fits that pattern.

I had met Amanda through a mutual friend, David Burnett of Students for Concealed Carry. SCC is the nation's preeminent grassroots organization fighting for the rights of law-abiding college students to be able to carry their firearms on campus. For some reason, state legislators, many governors and university officials across America continue to deny students, who otherwise meet the legal requirements, their constitutional right to carry their guns while on campus. Such is the case at the University of Nevada, Reno where fourth-year student Amanda Collins was prohibited from carrying her lawfully owned firearm. The same Nevada gun ban also forbids the keeping of a lawfully owned and carried gun anywhere inside a vehicle while on university property.

On Monday October 22nd, 2007 Amanda Collins played by the rules. On that same day, James Biela didn't give a *damn* about Nevada law.

This is her story.

"I WAS 22 YEARS OLD AND I WAS LIVING WITH SOME ROOM-mates about 20 minutes off campus. I was working and going to school and I was totally involved with my sorority. I was dating the man who is now my husband," she told me as we got started discussing the events that would change her life forever. "I was studying Secondary Education and English," she said. Working as a pre-k teacher, Amanda had her hands full with a classroom of 24, four- and five-year-olds.

A normal Monday morning, Amanda awoke to start her usual long day, which included teaching for half a day, studying and eventually taking a mid-term exam that night in her regular Monday evening class. "I probably woke up about 6:45 a.m. and got ready to go to work. It was during midterms so there's a higher level of stress. I left the house about 7:15 a.m. and was at work by 8 a.m. I had about 24 students on any given day," she said as we joked about having her hands full with the children. "It was a normal day," she chuckled as if somehow keeping control of two-dozen pre-k children was an easy task.

Leaving her job as scheduled at 1:00 p.m. when the afternoon teacher arrived, she took a drive over to her sorority house to have lunch with her sisters. "I had lunch and chatted with some of the girls about an upcoming meeting, then I went to my parents house to study for an upcoming midterm I had that evening in Teaching Literacy," she said. Studying intensely for the next few hours at her mom and dad's place, she eventually took off for class feeling good about her prospects on what was sure to be a challenging exam.

Leaving her parents house at 6:15 p.m. Amanda drove off for the university, called her boyfriend to let him know she was heading to the mid-term and told him that she would call him when she got home. "The leaves were changing and it's a beautiful drive so I was appreciating all of that," she recalled as she drove the 15 minutes from her parent's house to the university. She certainly had no reason to believe this night would be any different than any other Monday with the exception of the stress of the mid-term exam.

As she did every week, she pulled into the same covered parking garage she had always parked in, the very garage the campus police use to house their squad cars. "I parked on the ground floor. It has the ground floor and I think three floors above that. It's adjoined with the administration building and a cafeteria on the bottom of that building. It was directly across the way from where the College of Education is, which is where I was headed."

No stranger to self-defense, Amanda's father had taught her the safe use of firearms from the time she was five years old. Growing up around guns she was also a member of her high school rifle team. Schooled not only in the use of firearms from an early age, Amanda was also an expert in the martial arts. "My parents required my sister and me to get our second-degree black belts before we got our drivers licenses when we were 16," she told me. As part of her self-defense training Amanda was always very aware of her surroundings and was mindful of her own personal safety when she parked in the campus garage that Monday night. "I chose to park in that parking garage because I figured it would be better than walking across campus or off campus in the middle of the night when I got out of my class to get to my car," she said. Not only attentive to the distance of her walk back to the car, she was also parked in the same garage, on the same floor and less than 60 feet away from the visible campus police cruisers.

She did everything right.

Amanda grabbed her belongings, exited her car and took the short walk approximately 75 yards to her classroom building. Like the rest of her fellow students, she sat with other classmates discussing the impending mid-term exam they were about to take. Lasting three hours every Monday, her class tonight would keep the same schedule beginning at 7 p.m. and ending at 10 p.m. The mid-term occupied the first one and one half hours with a lecture following until the class adjourned. Feeling confident about the results of the test she had just taken, Amanda and three or four other students, all coeds who had parked in the same facility left the building together headed toward their vehicles.

"I left with a group of students, we all went together because there's a theory about safety in numbers," she remembered. "We were discussing the exam and comparing answers. We walked across the path and into the parking garage and I was the only one that parked on the ground floor. Everyone else had parked above me." As the other students got in an elevator and headed to their respective floors, Amanda continued to her own car. Using the techniques ingrained in her through her years of self-defense training, she remained alert as she neared her automobile. "As I approached my car I looked in and around my vehicle to see if there was anybody underneath just to check my surroundings and I was approaching it at a diagonal as I was taught to do through my martial arts training."

Alone, aware of her surroundings and looking for any possible dangers, she noticed a blue Dodge truck and a sedan parked across from her own vehicle but it's what she didn't see next that would alter the rest of her life.

"I didn't see the man who was hunched on the side of the truck with his feet where the wheel well is, and as I passed him he grabbed me from behind and um, I dropped everything I had been carrying, my binders and my keys and stuff." Ambushed from behind with no warning, James Biela grabbed Amanda, and violently forced her to the pavement. "The next thing I remember is him putting a metallic barrel, something very cold and hard against my temple and I knew, I just knew it was a firearm … and he clicked the safety off and told me not to say anything."

Familiar with firearms, Amanda had never been so petrified by the sound of a gun's safety before this night. What had always been a reassuring "click" in her hands over the years now took on an entirely different meaning. "The sound of a safety had never been so terrifying to me up until that moment. Up until that point it was always security," she said.

No more.

Now it represented a loaded firearm with a hair trigger pressed firmly and intentionally against her head in the hands of a madman, a maniac laying on top of her, holding her under his own weight on the floor of a parking garage late at night. "The whole time though, I wasn't afraid of the gun, I was afraid of the man who had the gun," she recalled.

Pinned to the floor of the parking garage next to her own vehicle and with a loaded firearm pressed firmly against her temple, Amanda Collins was brutally raped over the next 5-8 minutes. "I just went into survival mode. I kept telling myself it will be over soon … if I can just get through this," she said. "When he was finished he got up and pointed his gun at me and told me not to get up until he left." In what would then become a sick and defining moment exemplifying his utter depravity and ruthlessness, James Biela calmly complimented her on her attire before he bolted into the darkness and disappeared. "He informed me that he liked my skirt and thought it made me look good."

Staying on the ground until she could no longer hear his footsteps, Amanda Collins lay in shock and disbelief at what had just happened to her. Although her attacker had a hoodie pulled over his face for the duration of the assault, there was an instant according to Amanda, "that by the grace of God", she was able to get a good look at him even if for that brief moment, his face etched into her mind forever. "It was the face that burned into my memory and it was the face that haunted my nightmares." Amanda Collins had no idea just how important that split second of memory would become in the search for her attacker.

Scared and in shock, she wanted out of there. "I got up as quickly as possible, got in my vehicle, locked my doors and drove away," she noted. "In that moment it just seemed I did everything bad if I had ever found myself in that situation that I would have never done. I went to my sorority house and took a shower," a mere three blocks away from where she had been attacked moments earlier. After showering, Amanda slipped out of the house unnoticed by any of her sorority sisters and quietly departed for the home she shared with two other roommates in the city of Sparks, roughly 20 minutes away.

Shocked, in denial and disbelief, Amanda admits to not thinking clearly. Arriving home she went straight to bed. She remembers texting her boyfriend and "falling asleep I just convinced myself it was the worst nightmare I had ever had in my life and my brain just went into complete denial," she says reflecting back on the awful experience

Although Amanda had discussed the incident with her roommate over the course of the next few weeks, she herself had never called the police. Thinking it had been too long since the rape and feeling as if she had no evidence to file a report, it would be the case of a missing young woman and the action of her roommate that would eventually bring *her* case to the attention of law enforcement. Now January, three months since Amanda's brutal assault, Brianna Denison, a beautiful young 19-year-old woman had recently gone missing and would later be found murdered. Within one week of Brianna's disappearance, and without her prior knowledge, Amanda's roommate would notify law enforcement of the attack against her thinking it might have been the same person responsible for both crimes.

115

Amanda remembered, "They had gone to my work and I had already left for the day so my boss gave them my cell number and she called me to tell me some detectives had shown up looking for me. The next message was from the detective asking to meet with me." After speaking with detectives, she was still not convinced the cases were related but would soon find out that investigators had linked what happened to Brianna to a *second* victim who had been attacked in December, a mere two months after Amanda. Telling detectives that she had seen her attacker's face and with every reason now to believe the murder of Brianna and the attack against Amanda and the other victim were related, detectives asked her to provide details to their sketch artist. It was her vivid description from the memory seared into her brain the night of the rape that would provide the sketch used to snag James Biela during one of the largest manhunts in recent Nevada history as the community pulled together and searched for the serial rapist and murderer in their midst.

Eventually caught and charged one full year after the vicious attacks against Amanda, the second rape victim and for the murder of Brianna Dennison, ex-marine and pipe fitter, 28-year-old James Biela was tried and found guilty of three counts of rape, one count of kidnapping, one count of murder, and one count of assault with a deadly weapon. It was the assault with a deadly weapon charge that prosecutors attached for the attack against Amanda. Taking the stand and facing her attacker, Ms. Collins told him in front of a packed courtroom, "Though you didn't murder me, you killed the trusting and vivacious woman I was moments before you turned my world upside down."

116

Since that horrifying night in 2007, Amanda and her boyfriend have married and are raising a beautiful daughter together. With the assistance and support of her loving family and friends, Amanda took her story public. Along with the NRA and grassroots groups such as Students for Concealed Carry, she has dedicated herself to changing the laws that left her unable to defend herself on that fateful night. She has no doubts that if Nevada law had not disarmed her that evening, the second victim may never have been attacked and Brianna Denison may very well be alive.

Amanda has testified in front of the Nevada State Legislature in her tireless effort to change the law to allow good people to defend themselves against evil. Her story has appeared on national television, and she has been written about in newspaper articles and columns around the nation. She has appeared with me as a guest on Armed American Radio and continues the fight for gun rights. Following in the footsteps of others before her who have used their frightening experiences to make a difference in other people's lives, Amanda Collins is a true hero and American patriot.

James Biela was sentenced to death in June 2010 and is now sitting in a Nevada prison awaiting execution by lethal injection. For good measure, the judge tacked on an additional three consecutive life terms guaranteeing he would never walk free in the unlikely event of a successful appeal of his convictions and subsequent death sentence.

On the surface, she was doing everything right and shouldn't have become a victim. But in an ambush situation all that changes.

Chapter 14 - Ambushed and Alone

Rob Pincus

The Problem:

"**S**ITUATIONAL AWARENESS" IS OFTEN WORN LIKE A safety blanket by those with personal defense training, but sometimes provides little more than false confidence in the worst-case scenarios that we can face. After all, if your awareness works, you will avoid a fight or at least be somewhat ready for it when it comes, right?

In this case, Amanda was about as "ready" as anyone could imagine given her situation:

1. She had spent some number of years training in the martial arts.

2. She parked on the ground floor to minimize the time she spent in a danger area.

3. She left the building in a group and stayed with them as long as was practical.

4. She scanned the area of her car before approaching it.

On the surface, she was doing everything *right* and shouldn't have become a victim.

It's easy to say that she would've been safer if she had been carrying a gun, but I see no reason to think so. She was ambushed, knocked violently to the ground and had a gun placed to her head. That moment calls for fighting to control the attacker and his tool, and, only *then* considering using your own firearm. The presence of a gun would not likely have helped her in the moment of her particular attack.

As you get ready to read the next two sections of this chapter, keep in mind what I said in my introduction: Playing "Monday Morning Quarterback" is never emotionally comfortable, especially when reviewing incidents like this one. But, analyzing what has happened before, picking out the important lessons and looking at what could have gone differently is the whole reason for this work.

Change the Story:

IF ANY OF THOSE STEPS HAD BEEN SIGNIFICANTLY DIFFERENT, the story may have turned out very differently as well:

1. If Amanda had actually trained in practical defensive skills, and not traditional children's martial arts, she might have had options when she found herself on the ground with an attacker who was focusing on more than just protecting himself as he completed the sexual assault. She might also have had intuitive level protective skills that might have kicked in when she was first grabbed. If we add a

gun to the equation, then a very specialized course like *Extreme Close Quarters Tactics* or Craig Douglas' *Extreme Close Quarters Concepts* might have given her the confidence and skillset required to deal with gaining control of the bad guy's gun and using her own while in contact with her threat.

2. If Amanda had car-pooled that night, she almost certainly wouldn't have been attacked. Similarly, if she had parked in a slightly less "text-book-safe" area with her other classmates, she would've been able to avoid isolation.

3. If her friends had been compelled to walk Amanda to her car and then continued on in their own group, Amanda also would've been able to avoid isolation. People should be less shy about asking for such a small inconvenience and/or quicker to offer it to those, especially women, who are going to break off from a group for a walk to a car or home.

4. Ultimately, there is no way to be completely sure that you aren't walking into a trap, but looking past the quick scan to think about areas where someone could be hiding can increase the likelihood of finding anyone lying in wait. One thing that can be done relatively easily is to walk past your intended destination, changing the predicted route to your car or door. Doing this will often foil the plan of anyone planning an ambush. It doesn't mean that you won't be attacked, of course, but it may allow you some level of warning that can increase your

practical readiness to defend yourself.

Training and Preparation:

Let's take a look at how the steps Amanda took failed to protect her:

1. There is a vast difference between 99% of the "martial arts" being taught to children and practical unarmed defensive training. Unfortunately, not all martial arts instructors are clear about the differences and can facilitate a false confidence in one's ability to protect one's self. When you are looking for unarmed defensive skills for yourself or your children, look for courses that teach fighting, not kata, counting in foreign languages, the importance of rituals and/or "life lessons" of hard work, integrity, honor and respect … some programs teach those things *along with* self defense, but they are rare.

2. Bad guys are looking for victims and they know the same cliché's that we do … park under the lights, walk in groups, hold your keys in your hand as you approach your vehicle. If you are following conventional wisdom about how to remain safe, you need to be aware that the bad guy might be very well aware of your "safety trick" and be working to undermine it, or even take advantage of it. The specific circumstances of your situation will dictate how to best increase your odds, not relying on generalizations and what are possibly no more than myths. In Amanda's case, planning ahead to

park in the same area (and at the same time) as her classmates, even if it was on the top floor or in a dark area, probably would've been a better choice. As we have discussed already, isolation, no matter how brief, is one of the bad guy's most sought after things. Carpooling is another great option to keep yourself from being isolated.

3. Overwhelmingly, the worst-case scenarios that people face when it comes to personal attacks are defined as "ambushes". They are unexpected and sudden. No matter how "aware" you think you are, there are going to be holes in your focus. Blind spots, distractions, danger areas, things *requiring* your attention and misdirection are all part of our everyday lives. Too much of our training and thought about personal defense is approached from an in-control perspective. For years, I have preached the importance of being open to the idea that you can get caught off guard and be required to fight from a position just like the one that Amanda found herself in: Already grabbed, already on our back and already with a lethal tool being used against us. This is a very different situation than being "aware" of a potential threat, going to a ready position and scanning quickly for additional threats before focusing on the bad guy and issuing a verbal command. I thought this topic was so important, in fact, that I wrote a whole book about it in 2012, titled *Counter Ambush*.

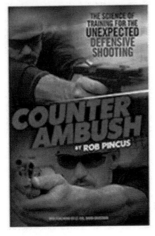

Counter Ambush from Rob Pincus is a thorough exploration of both WHY and HOW you should structure your personal defense training to deal with a worst-case scenario ambush situation. *Counter Ambush* is thoroughly supported by over twenty years of research and training in the area of training for all levels of personal defense: Military, Law Enforcement, Security or the Responsible Individual.

Sections include:

-Understanding the need for Counter Ambush Training

-Neuroscience of Counter Ambush Training

-Physiology of Counter Ambush Training

-The Physics of Intuitive Defensive Shooting

-Developing your Counter Ambush Training Program

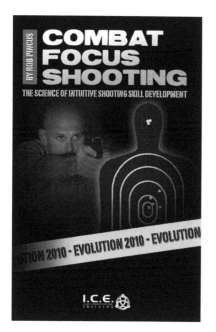

Combat Focus Shooting: The Science of Intuitive Shooting Skill Development is the cutting edge of understanding how to quickly gain lifesaving firearms skills regardless of your experience, background or the context of your firearms use. Based on working well with what your body does naturally during a dynamic critical incident and focusing on the concept of the balance of speed and precision, this program doesn't just tell you what to do; it explains *why*. This is not just another tool for your toolbox; *Combat Focus® Shooting is the best information the author and his team of instructors have to offer.*

That life-changing moment can come at any time. When it happens will you be ready to spring into action? Do you have a plan? What will you do?

Chapter 15 - In the Blink of an Eye

Mark Walters

IT CAN HAPPEN ANYWHERE, IT CAN HAPPEN ANYTIME, AND I can assure you that when it does it will happen at break-neck speed. We tell this as a reminder that life-altering events come in many forms and in many shapes, but I was reminded during a past family vacation just how fast life can change and how you had better be mentally prepared for the instant, and I do mean the instant, that it may occur.

My family took a summer vacation a few years back and we found ourselves in Myrtle Beach, South Carolina with in-laws, brothers and sisters, and cousins, etc., the entire crew, if you will. Typical of over-crowded tourist destinations, Myrtle Beach is loaded with packed restaurants and filled to the brim with tourist-trap shops full of, well … tourists being trapped into buying things they would never normally buy at home. You know, little shot glasses and mugs with their names on them and the like, silly henna tattoos and stupid hats they will never wear again.

Something as simple as deciding where to eat when you're with fifteen people is a chore unto itself, and it was eventually settled one particular evening that we would be having dinner at a decent, local seafood restaurant near a boardwalk along the main drag somewhere. Afterward, the plan was to hit the tourist shops, and, as a single member of a large group, who was I to suggest otherwise? Upon leaving the seafood restaurant, I was trailing behind my five-year-old son as we crossed a little street leading to the "strip of traps" with the rest of the family meandering just up ahead.

That is when I heard someone's voice ring out from among the dozens of shoppers and tourists crossing that little walkway to and from the shops, "Oh, my God! That little boy is choking! SOMEBODY DO SOMETHING!" Now anyone who knows me will tell you that choking is one of my biggest phobias. I don't know why it is – it just is – and it has been since I was a kid. I don't have any recollection of anything traumatic regarding a choking incident occurring in my life, and I have even asked my parents if something had happened that would give me this life-long phobia. With the exception of my younger sister getting smacked in the back a few times to cough up a chicken bone in a cabin during a fishing trip to Northern Michigan when we were very young, I can't really pinpoint an episode that would have had an impact on me. Heck, I remember thinking the incident with my sister was funny.

The fact is that the thought of choking scares me to death when it comes to my own children and the fear that I may not

128

be around, or be in the shower, or driving down the road if it were to happen just freaks me out. I hate it, but in a weird kind of way, because of my fear, I guess the thought of it occurring to one of my kids is never really too far from my mind, even if I am not consciously thinking about it at that exact moment.

Here came that moment when I was least expecting it.

Hearing that woman's desperate voice, I glanced down nonchalantly not even thinking it could be one of my children in danger, I mean it never happens to us right? That's when I saw my son stopped in the middle of the road, bent over and leaning, almost falling forward. He appeared unable to breath or even make a sound. I immediately, without hesitation, without even thinking, without batting an eyelid, without freaking out, dove down to one knee behind him, reached my arms around him, and forced him upright. Placing my hands in the Heimlich positions, I began to steadily pull inward and upward. Failure was not an option. It HAD to work! I never thought otherwise … It just HAD to! Thank God it did.

On the third pull, he made a coughing sound and up came half of one of those round peppermint candies that just minutes earlier I had said he could eat when he reached into the bowl on the cash register counter as we exited the restaurant. As a result of that damned piece of candy – that innocent piece of peppermint candy that all of us have eaten at some point in our lives – there I was, standing in the crowded intersection trying to keep my son from dying right there in the street.

After it came out of his throat and fell to the street he stood motionless for a couple of seconds, caught his breath, and then began to cry loudly. He ran to his mother after he caught his breath and jumped into her arms. When I walked over and began rubbing his back, I heard him ask, "Am I going to get sick now?" I heard some clapping, and glancing around, noticed that everyone who had been walking by had stopped to watch, almost in fascination, you know, the car wreck thing. Rubbernecking. The "better you than me" syndrome.

> Eighty percent of choking victims are younger than five years old.

Some people, complete strangers, had begun to clap when they realized he was going to be okay. It was extremely frightening, to say the least, and it took me a couple of seconds to realize what had just occurred. I paced in a circle for a minute thinking about the magnitude of what might have happened had I not been there. Would someone else have stepped up to the plate? Would someone with no emotional connection to my little son have done the same thing I did by diving to help save his life? Would they be fearful of being sued and let a little boy choke to death in front of their eyes as they stood there while talking to a 911 operator? I don't know. I know what I would like to think, but I can't be sure. Not in today's world. I can only be thankful that I was there to help him and not think about what would have happened had I been absent at that exact moment.

The entire scary episode unleashed itself in a split second. One moment I was taking a stroll, thinking about the fact that I had eaten too much dinner, needed an Alka Seltzer and never wanted to eat food again in my entire adult life when – wham! There I was, in the blink of an eye, on my knees pulling a life-saving technique I had never used before, on my little son. No time to think, only time to react. No time to question myself, only time to act. No time to ask for assistance, only time to immediately take charge on my own. No time to get scared, only time to fix the problem, a problem that could have killed my son ... and time was running out, quickly. I had no time to do anything but REACT to a situation I did not ask for, never want to be in again, and wouldn't wish on anyone else. I'm not afraid to tell you that it was terrifying.

> **Over 17,000 infants and children are treated for choking every year.**

It dawned on me later that evening, as I reflected on what had happened and what might have happened; life can and does change instantly, and usually does so without warning: a heart attack, a car wreck, a fall, a violent crime. Just like that, in a snap, in an instant, when you are least expecting it and it will come out of nowhere, wham, there you are fighting for your life or the lives of your loved ones or maybe even an innocent bystander. One moment you are talking to your friend about where you are going next after dinner, and the next second your friend is lying on the ground and his attacker is turning his attention on you. Are YOU ready for it?

Like me, you may have had similar events in your own life that have impacted your future actions. Maybe you have been in an auto accident or a near miss, for that matter. Maybe you have been a victim of a violent crime, had a brush with a sickness or other health scare, or some other threatening situation. Like me, you have learned from these events in your life – hopefully! As a result of incidents like these that we all face in our daily lives, I am a HUGE proponent of always being prepared, always being aware of your surroundings, and always having a plan of action.

This does not mean that you must walk around like a zombie with your eyes wide open in an unblinking stare, your mind filled with "what if" scenarios as your children are eating, or carrying a medical kit over your shoulder "just in case." As renowned firearms trainer and co-author of this work, Rob Pincus once said, "Being prepared doesn't mean ordering from a Braille menu so you don't have to take your eyes off of the front door," but it does mean to be thinking in advance of what could happen and to simply have a plan in the event it does. It's why you have health insurance; it's why you have auto insurance; it's why you have a fire extinguisher, and it's why you took that CPR class. It's why you have food in your pantry and gas in your car, and it's why you carry a gun for your own protection … just in case.

How do I perform the Heimlich Maneuver?

Also called "Abdominal Thrusts" the Heimlich maneuver can be performed safely on both children and adults, though it isn't recommended for use on infants less than 1 year old. It is also possible to perform the maneuver on yourself.

- For a sitting or standing person who is conscious, position yourself behind them and reach your arms around the choking person's waist.
- Place your fist, thumb side in, just above the person's navel and grab the fist tightly with your other hand.
- Pull your fist abruptly upward and inward to increase airway pressure behind the obstructing object and force it from the windpipe.
- If the person is conscious and lying on his or her back, straddle the person facing the head. Push your grasped fist upward and inward in a maneuver similar to the one above.

The above procedure may need to be repeated several times before the foreign object is dislodged.

... your worst-case scenario moment isn't likely to phone in a warning ahead of time.

Chapter 16 - The Worst Moment

Rob Pincus

<u>The Problem:</u>

THERE WILL BE NO WARNING FOR THE WORST MOMENT OF your life. There is nothing that Mark could have done, short of feeding his son intravenously and making him wear a "Jason Mask" all the time, that could have prevented his son from choking on that piece of candy. Kids eat things, things sometimes get caught the wrong way in kid's throats... tragically, some number of kids die from this every year. If it is a newborn choking in its sleep because it was left on it's back or 1 year old choking on coins left as toys in its crib, we are talking about something entirely different... but, there is simply no practical way to ensure that a child (or an adult, for the matter!) won't at some point in their lives choke on food.

Choking on food is like getting attacked while walking through a parking garage and getting grabbed from behind a car. Choking on food is like having someone you trust give you a ride on a cold night, then pull out a gun and shoot at you. Choking on food is like having two people walk into a public bathroom and rob you. Bad things can happen at any time, regardless of your preparation.

Change the Story:

In this case, everything worked out very well in our story ... so, we're going to change it for the worse.

What if Mark had not been aware of the dangers of choking? What if he had not had a respectful awareness of the threat that the possibility of choking poses? Obviously, his son may have died that night. Or his son's brain may have gone without oxygen for so long while he was waiting for medical assistance that he suffered permanent brain damage. At best, Mark and his son would've been left in the street *hoping* that someone who was prepared and trained to deal with that situation came to their rescue.

> But what happens if everything doesn't go right? What then?

Sadly, this is the situation that many Americans find themselves in every day when it comes to some very real possible dangers: armed robbery, assaults, rapes and murders are all possibilities that we face every day.

Training and Preparation:

Luckily, like choking deaths, they are relatively rare.... but, they are also just as real. They deserve some portion of our attention. Knowing basic responses to choking is something that our society has taken seriously for a few decades. We all learn the Heimlich Maneuver, we've all seen countless posters in public spaces with the proper steps to take if someone if choking. We need to take personal defense just as seriously. I don't need to quote statistics for us to know that the incidents of choking deaths in restaurants dropped significantly once training was common and choking response posters were made common. I have no doubt that the same effect would be seen in regard to violent crime if more people were trained and prepared for personal defense and if discussions about it were more common. If posters in every convenience store reminded everyone to find a clear lane of fire before shooting at an armed robber, my guess is that armed robberies would decrease!

> Gear your training towards developing intuitive, recognition level, skills.

The other important lesson to learn from Mark's story is that your worst-case scenario moment isn't likely to phone in a warning ahead of time. All of your training and preparation should be geared towards developing intuitive *recognition level* skills just like Mark had that night in the street. He didn't have to think; he didn't have to stretch out; he didn't have to get into some specific position, and he didn't recognize "pre-contact cues" nor did his awareness allow him to see the threat coming. Mark **observed** something that his brain **reacted** to the stimulus by focusing on it. Because of his previous training and thought, he **recognized** what was happening and he *responded* properly. This

137

ORRR Loop (an evolution of Col. Boyd's O.O.D.A. Loop) should be the goal of all of your training and practice. You don't want to have to analyze the information coming into your brain and then have to make complex decisions about what to do. If you train realistically and frequently, you should be able recognize what you need to do and respond intuitively, using as little time, effort and energy as possible.

Here are some helpful statistics.

DEATH BY CHOKING IS PREVALENT IN CHILDREN UNDER AGE four due to a small airway, natural curiosity, oral fixation, and incomplete chewing. According to statistics from the Centers for Disease Control and Prevention, choking rates in 2001 were highest in infants.

The following foods are commonly considered choking hazards:
- hot dogs
- hard candy
- chewing gum
- nuts and seeds
- chunks of meat or cheese
- whole grapes
- popcorn
- chunks of peanut butter
- raw vegetables
- raisins

The following objects are commonly considered choking hazards:

- coins
- buttons
- marbles
- small balls
- deflated balloons
- watch batteries
- jewelry
- ball point pen caps and paper clips
- arts and crafts supplies
- small toys and toys with small detachable parts

The bottom line is this: Be especially careful with children. Watch what they put in their mouth. It's a life or death issue.

Mark's Final Thoughts

Transferring the words of crime victims to paper from an interview is never easy. The pain and suffering in their voices or the faraway look in their eyes as they recall the events that forever changed their lives is difficult to explain and even harder to convey in print. It is palpable. It is frightening and it resonates with me as a human being. I hope it resonated with you. I genuinely feel for these fine people and empathize with them as they recalled for me the events that undeniably made them who they are today. By allowing you the opportunity to read their stories, these good people are hoping that we all learn from their suffering and fear. In each case I have been told the same thing in one way or another, "I hope someone can learn from my experience."

Will you?

It's not easy. I'll be the first to admit it. It is not easy to make a decision to be prepared every day. It is difficult to do and it requires you to be "on" virtually every waking minute of your life. You must be able to look yourself in the mirror and ask yourself some very difficult questions. Do you have what it takes to be prepared, every minute of every day when life's pitcher throws you the inevitable curveball when you least expect it? Are you willing to seek the training, incur the costs and give the time necessary to live a life prepared for the inevitable? Are you capable of putting a gun in your purse or wearing a holster every day? Are you capable of admitting that life can be cruel and that evil does in fact exist? Are you willing to take the steps necessary to face it?

Are you willing to prevail?

The people you read about and the experiences they shared with you are hopefully a wake up call. Hopefully they are a real life reminder that your own mortality will show itself when you least expect it and although the risk of criminal attack is extremely low, will you let their experience be your guide?

I asked the question above, are you willing to prevail? The sad fact is that you may not be able to escape if evil chooses to visit you at a time and place of its choosing, and sadly you may not be able to survive the encounter. However, one thing is certain ... Your failure to prepare will guarantee the outcome.

Will you choose to refuse to be a victim?

Mark Walters

Rob's Final Thoughts

Now that you've read these stories and our thoughts on them and the lessons to be learned from them, what are your "take-aways"?   What do you think are the most valuable things you got from this book and the process you went through reading it?

- Will you change your behavior?
- Will you change the places you live, work or spend free time?
- Will you spend time with different people?
- Will you buy a new piece of equipment?
- Will you take a class?
- Will you talk to those whom you care for about this book?

For some of you the answer to all of those questions will hopefully be "yes". Other readers will not find themselves needing changes in every area, and will answer "yes" to fewer questions. Maybe you will only answer "yes" to the last one … and then your friend or family member may make changes in their lives that make them safer.

Life is full of changes, the best ones come from the experience of learning. Making a conscious decision to change your life in some way to make it better because you gained knowledge is the best way to take control of your life.

Aside from the big picture take-aways, remember that this book is not about carrying a gun with you at all times. That would be a gross over-simplification of the issues that I hope we brought to your attention. Personal defense is about much more than any one tool. Your behavior, your mindset, your awareness, your planning, your ability to think critically and make decisions rapidly and, ultimately, your ability to defend yourself physically (with or without any tools) are all a vital part of staying safe.

Personally, I look forward to hearing from readers and finding out exactly what you took away from this book ... so send me an email and let me know!

Train Well!

– Rob Pincus
rob@icetraining.us

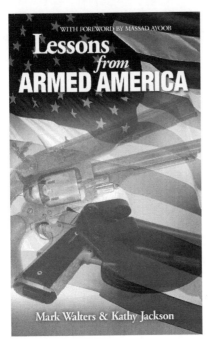

Whether you are new to the concept of armed defense or have long since made it a part of a prudent lifestyle, you'll find much that is useful in this book. Read it the way Kathy and Mark wrote it, that is, don't just look at it, but study it for its lessons! – Massad Ayoob Founder, Lethal Force Institute Author of *In the Gravest Extreme* –

These are serious words from Massad, the Master of self defense! Don't rely on others to protect yourself and your loved ones. "Lessons from Armed America" is the essential primer for self defense. Kathy and Mark are the experts that answer all your questions on stalking, real-life firefights, prevention and awareness, as well as carjacking and use of nonlethal force. They tell it like it is with candor and compassion, speaking through both experience and well-thought-out-research. If you're serious about protecting your family, this is the one book you MUST read!

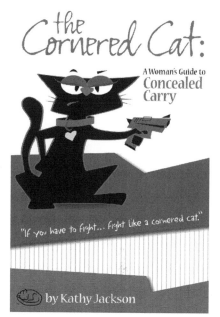

The Cornered Cat is the ultimate resource for women who choose to carry a firearm for self defense. It covers everything from cleaning a pistol to methods of carry. It tells women everything they ever wanted to know about how to carry a firearm for self defense. The Cornered Cat is all about women that have chosen or are considering choosing firearms for self defense, sport, or just wanting to understand more about what their menfolk find so fascinating. This book contains a wealth of information presented in Kathy's warm and often humorous style. She tackles the serious considerations of using deadly force in defense of oneself and loved ones in a thought-provoking, non-judgmental, "between girlfriends" prose that is neither threatening nor sugar-coated, just very real.

Order anywhere books are sold!

In Memory of and Deep Appreciation

I offer this separate dedication on a very deep and personal level to former Ohio State Representative, Michael DeBose from Cleveland, Ohio and his family. Rep. DeBose's story appeared as the chapter, *The Political Bravery of Michael DeBose* in *Lessons from Armed America*, with Kathy Jackson. He had voted against Ohio's Concealed Carry legislation twice before changing his mind about armed self-defense and subsequently changing his vote in favor after becoming a victim of an armed assault while strolling through his neighborhood on an afternoon walk. I reached out to him after reading his story in the *Cleveland Plain Dealer* and he granted me an extensive interview. He wanted his story in print and later would became a vocal and public advocate for the right to bear arms, challenging his own party line. The two of us developed a unique bond and a quick friendship that saw him calling me "just to say hello", to wish my family a "happy Thanksgiving, or seek advice on a choice of carry gun. Representative Michael DeBose passed away on April 23, 2012 of complications from Parkinson's disease at the young age of 58. Although it took a life-threatning experience for him to understand the right to bear arms for self-defense, Michael DeBose exhibited incredible strength and courage standing up to the political forces within the vehemently anti-gun forces of his own party and a rabidly anti-gun local media. He is evidence that the right to bear arms knows no boundaries, be they political, racial or economic and that we all share the basic human right to defend our lives. He is missed.

– Mark Walters

Appendix I - School Shootings

Mark Walters

A Short and Painful Lesson

SHARI THORNBURG WAS A SANDY HOOK ELEMENTARY School staffer when Newtown, Connecticut resident Adam Lanza walked into the school on the morning of December 14th, 2012 and opened fire murdering 26 people including 20 small children. In a *USA Today* column, *"School shooting survivor tells her story"* (*USA Today,* 9:37 am EST December 19th, 2012) written as part of an ongoing series titled, *"Connecticut School Shooting Victims,"* Ms. Thornburg is quoted extensively about the day of the killings and her experience inside the school.

According to the December 19th story, having just been "buzzed-in" through the locked doors, Ms. Thornburg walked into the principals office to "sign in" and begin her work day as an "assistant to a 4th grader with special needs." Walking down the hallway into a math-science room to drop off her personal belongings and after a brief conversation with two other staffers, she said, "Then we heard pop-pop-pop, pop-pop-pop, and I thought, 'That's a weird noise.' I first thought it was the janitor taking down risers and setting up tables."

Ms. Thornburg's discussion with *USA Today* is extremely important as her account puts us inside the mayhem and gives us the perspective of someone who did the only thing she could do at that moment in time, and while defenseless in the classic sense, survived the gruesome attack. She continued telling *USA Today* that she heard "more shots, screaming, crying and whimpering." According to her account, she and the two other staffers that she was talking with at the moment the shooting started had locked themselves into the teacher's room "and the three of us struggled to get in a small closet."

The following statements she gave to the *USA Today* in that December 19th, 2012 piece open a window of opportunity for us to paint a vivid picture inside our minds eye of what being in that school would have been like. After you read her statements, close your eyes, envision the school you attended as a child, feel the concrete blocks as you drag your hands down the walls walking to class, see the painted murals in the hallways depicting a current event of the day and smell the cafeteria food. Try to imagine how the concrete blocks of the hallways and classrooms would echo the sounds of ricocheting gunfire as you cowered in fear for your life, unprotected under a desk or locked behind a closed door, unable to run.

Imagine this:

"We heard everything over the intercom, though it was muffled because our closet door was closed."

"We just waited in the closet, saying The Lord's Prayer out loud over and over and over again, and praying for all staff members and the children."

The janitor's screams of "Put the gun down, put the gun down."

"It was scary when we heard the classroom door jiggle and thought it was the gunman. When the shooting was over, we learned it was the janitor checking to see whether the door was locked."

According to her account, one of the rooms bypassed by the shooter was a classroom filled with first-graders, and in it "Teacher, Kaitlin Roig, had piled 16 first-graders on top of one another in the bathroom."

In probably her most telling statement of all, a topic I talk about on the air on a frequent basis, our ability as human beings to deny evil's existence becomes painfully apparent when she is quoted, *"Who would have thought this would happen in an idyllic little school in the woods where you would want your kids to go?"*

No matter how many years shall pass since Sandy Hook, December 14th, 2012 will remain one of America's darkest days, much like our recollections of Columbine. On that tragic afternoon in April of 1999, monsters Eric Harris and Dylan Klebold wreaked death and destruction on their fellow students at Columbine High School in Littleton, Colorado killing 12 fellow students and a beloved coach. The evil cowards also took their own lives.

I refer back to Columbine for there is still very much to be learned in the years since that awful day. The experiences of the murdered students as recollected by the survivors continue to provide us a glimpse inside the "gun free, safety zone" when evil decides to act. While much has been written about the Columbine victims since 1999, when an event such as Sandy Hook and other school shootings occur years later, it may be wise to revisit those past experiences for comparisons to similarities as we search for answers today...and wonder aloud why we continue to allow our children to remain vulnerable.

As I remind you of these past events, please keep in mind the statements of Shari Thornburg as she and her colleagues huddled in fear, defenseless and at the mercy of pure evil while it acted in a gun free, killing zone many years later.

Brian Anderson was a 17-year-old student who had just walked past Klebold and Harris. He noticed they had guns but thought they were toy props when he was fired upon. With other students and a teacher, he retreated to the library and took refuge in a storage room and huddled behind a locked door, defenseless and at the mercy of evil.

Brian survived that day.

17 year-old Cassie Bernall wouldn't be so lucky. Like many other students in the library that day, she had taken to the floor seeking safety under a desk with another student after teacher Patti Nielson began screaming for students to "Get down." Cassie became known for her supposed response to an alleged question asked by one of the killers' seconds before taking her life. As the story goes, Eric Harris slapped the top of the desk she was cowering under and hauntingly looked below it yelling "Peek-a-boo" before asking her if she believed in God. She was shot after supposedly answering "Yes." No one knows for sure if the actual events unfolded that way, however there is no disputing that she was shot in the head at point-blank range with Eric Harris's sawed-off shotgun, instantly ending her promising young life in a horrifying way.

Corey DePooter was another 17 year-old student who found himself in the library on that fateful day. Also hiding under a table like other defenseless students and teachers, Dylan Klebold would soon take aim at him. Firing multiple times, Klebold coldly murdered Corey with a barrage of gunfire hitting him with multiple shots in his upper body, killing him instantly.

I could continue to go down the heartbreaking list of victims and the scenarios they found themselves in before being murdered but I don't believe it's necessary. The fact of the matter is that these stories are hauntingly similar, regardless of where they geographically occur and at what time in history. The teachers and students names at each event, whether it is Columbine, Virginia Tech or Sandy Hook Elementary could easily be swapped with one another. Whether they were survivors or murder victims, the results would be the same; defenseless schools full of defenseless administrators and by default, defenseless children in a killing zone.

These horrifying stories force us to ask ourselves some deep questions, not the least of which is how we continue to allow our most precious assets, our children, to remain vulnerable in the very places they should be the safest when not in the presence of their families, their schools.

The hard fact is that the majority of our nations schools remain phony *gun-free* zones designed to placate the gun-hating politicians who would send their own children to private school with private security while doing nothing to stop criminals who break our laws. Until we can remedy the problem for the sake of the safety of our nations children we must ask, does being disarmed by law in our schools necessarily mean we must remain *defenseless?*

Rob Pincus

The Problem:

SCHOOL ATTACKS ARE AN ABOMINATION. UNFORTUNATELY, it has become apparent that there are people so deranged that they will show up at a school intent on killing children. We also know that other predators will seek out similar "gun-free zones" to wreak havoc and to prey on those whom they assume will be both unable and unwilling to defend themselves. No amount of hoping, posturing, screening, profiling or vigilant awareness will prevent these atrocities.

Still, there are those in our society who continue to ignore the reality of school attacks and our need to plan and to deal with them in a practical way. These people exist on both sides of the gun-control issue. On the pro-gun side, too many people reduce the issue to "arm the teachers!" ignoring the simple fact that teachers need to be focused on educating, not on security. Many teachers are unfamiliar with firearms and simply would not be comfortable being armed. Similarly, many of the teachers who would be comfortable with being armed have not been trained to do so professionally in an environment like a school. On the other side of the gun issue, are people who honestly believe that posting a sign that says "no guns allowed" is actually meaningful to a psychotic murderer. That kind of naïveté is the same mindset that puts policies in place amounting to little more than "hide and hope" in our nation's schools.

The prevailing policy for responding to school attackers in the United States over the last decade has been "Lockdown". While there are subtle variations, the key components of a lockdown policy are to get students out of the halls and into a classroom, to lock the door and draw the shades (if possible), huddle the kids out of view of the doors/windows (if possible) and wait for help to arrive. Again, I refer to these as "Hide and Hope" strategies. They amount to a coin toss for the students and teachers: If the bad guy gets to them before the police are able to respond and stop him, they are left as victims.

Change the Story

IN THE PAST, WE'VE LEARNED THAT WHEN SCHOOL ATTACKERS have actually been confronted, they have almost always been stopped. This has been true even in cases where those resisting were not armed with guns. While there are exceptions, it can certainly be said that when spree attackers in a densely populated area have not been confronted, they simply continue to hurt and kill with impunity.

Students, teachers and others who spend their days in areas that may be targeted by a spree killer need to be given other options. They need to be empowered to do more than just wait to be rescued when they are faced with evil.

Training and Preparation

ON THE AFTERNOON OF THE TRAGEDY AT SANDY HOOK, I WAS asked by a student what I thought they should tell their children when they got home from school. I thought for quite a while before responding and ended up writing a short article so that my response could be shared with others. Within a few days, that article grew into a course outline for students and teachers, and I taught a two-hour seminar for kids from the ages of about 10 to 17 in my hometown. The short program was a modified version of things we teach people for home and unarmed defense, adjusted for the context of a school attack. Over the course of a couple of weeks, that seminar evolved into the School Attacker Response Course (SARC).

Here is the initial article that I wrote:

1. Let's remember that these events are INCREDIBLY RARE. This event, and those like it will be talked about for decades. How many people today have mentioned "Columbine" ? That was over a decade ago. How about "Beslan" ? That was almost a decade ago. Pennsylvania one-room schoolhouse" ? Over six years ago. The reason we reference incidents from the past is that these attacks are far from common and they are incredibly sensationalized because of the emotional components of the scale of the tragedy. It cannot be ignored that the politics of gun control also fuel the sensationalism and our communal memory formation of the event. I would stress educating your kids about the incredibly low likelihood that they will ever be touched by this kind of violence at their school.

2. Empower your children with a plan.

I will use the concepts that we teach as the fundamental responses for home defense:

EVADE: If you hear or see shooting at your school: GET AWAY. Go around as many corners or behind as many doors as you can. Don't forget to mention windows and the fact that a one-story drop may not be a big deal if the bad guy is about to break through the door.

HIDE/BARRICADE: Get out of the way and out of sight. Lock and/or block doors, if you can. "Hiding" might be as simple as remaining still and quiet in the corner of a room with a locked door (a corner that can't been seen through any window in the doorway).

ARM YOURSELF: Obviously, this isn't going to mean a gun. It could mean a fire extinguisher, a chair, a heavy book, a bat, a broom, a bucket, scissors … virtually anything. Get the thought process going and have your kids think about the things in their classroom that they could use as defensive tools. Remind them that they might need to point out these tools to the teacher in the room.

COMMUNICATE: If there is a cell phone there, make sure that they contact the police. After that, they should be encouraged to contact you … so long as talking won't reveal their position.

RESPOND AS APPROPRIATE: Tell your children to fight. Tell them to do whatever they can to survive. Tell them to recruit others in the effort and, if nothing else, swarm the bad guy. It has been demonstrated that pleading for mercy or "remaining still" and "hoping" are not effective methods for survival in these situations.

3. Keep the politics to a minimum, but prepare them for the fact that some misguided people might blame the tools of the murderer instead of the murderer. Children, especially scared or confused children, are easily influenced. Depending on their age,

they may be forming opinions that they will hold for the rest of their lives. Their education is your responsibility. Encourage them to be critical thinkers and apply logic to the question of what/who to blame, not emotion.

As the School Attacker Response Course (SARC) developed, the process that we advocated was streamlined:

1. Evade: Get away from the attacker, or out of range of the attack.

2. Barricade: Make it harder for the attacker to reach you.

3. Respond: If the attacker reaches you, use any improvised defensive tool, including your body, to defend yourself.

In the months that have followed, I.C.E. Training Company has conducted SARC Instructor Certification opportunities across the country from Florida to California, and our instructors have taught seminars in every region of the country as well. SARC programs (including instructor courses) are taught 100% free of charge. I.C.E. Training Company is underwriting all expenses to get this program into as many schools as possible. There have also been other examples of similar programs springing up around the country. Many school systems are quickly evolving their approach to these situations from the hide and hope to more proactive strategies.

After the Columbine school killings in the late 1990s, the law enforcement community had to evolve their response to school attacks. For the preceding two decades, more and more agencies had basically issued orders to patrol officers to establish a perimeter around those types of incidents and wait for the SWAT Teams (officers with better equipment and training) to arrive. Essentially, this was a police version of "hide and hope". Over the last decade, those policies have been largely eradicated. It is vital that the failed lockdown policies are removed from our schools as soon as possible and replaced with programs that actually empower people to not simply wait for those with better equipment and training to save them. I feel strongly that teaching children age-appropriate versions of Evade-Barricade-Respond throughout their school years, and including drills and scenario training in the same way that we do with Fire Response Plans, will have dramatic effects on the next generation's understanding of their right and responsibility to self-defense. The institution of defensive training for students could have profound effects on the reduction of problems with bullying and other types of assaults as well. If we teach kids that they can (and should!) take action when they are threatened with violence, I believe they will become more responsible citizens and better able to take care of themselves in general.

To receive more information on the School Attacker Response Course go to www.schoolattackerresponse.com.

Appendix II - Defensive Handgun Choice

Excerpt from the book *Counter Ambush*. Reprinted with permission of the author, Rob Pincus.

I'm going to give you some tangible, objective information that you can use at the range and your local gun shop about the physics of counter ambush shooting and gun handling. This will be particularly applicable to the context of a DCI. The first thing that you need to consider is the fit of your firearm. First and foremost, the firearm has to fit your hand. If the firearm that you're going to use to defend yourself doesn't fit well in your hand, you're going to have to work harder than you should need to in order to use it.

First, you want to make sure you can get a good, full grip on the firearm. You need to be able to have the web of your hand (between the thumb and index finger) directly behind the gun so that your thumb knuckle is beside the gun, not under the back of the frame. The axis of the movement of the slide should be aligned with your wrist when you are at extension. Make sure that your index finger can comfortably reach the trigger while your hand is in this position. Much discussion occurs about the best connection between your trigger finger and the trigger, but you really shouldn't over-think it. For defensive shooting, anywhere on the pad of the tip of your finger is good (If it is the inward half of the pad, all the better).

You want to make sure that you can hold the firearm so that there's no gap above your hand, relative to the top of the grip area, in order to help you manage recoil. That's also going to be important to the physics of the gun being reliable and for you to deliver a rapid string of fire efficiently.

Unfortunately, if you head to any public range, you will see some people cheating their hand one way or the other so that they can reach the trigger, which puts them in a bad physical relationship to the gun, which indicates that the gun doesn't fit their hand. There are so many guns available in so many shapes and sizes that it's ridiculous for any adult with a fully formed and functioning hand to have to compromise fit. Many of the recommended defensive firearms even have different sizes within one model line or interchangeable grips to make them customizeable to the owner.

It is important to acknowledge some people are forced to carry a specific firearm. If you're in the military, law enforcement, in a particular line of private security work, or possibly on a very limited budget, you may not have the option of switching from one gun to another. When someone comes to a two or three-day defensive shooting class, they are spending a lot of money. In some cases, thousands of dollars are spent to be there: tuition, ammunition, travel, food, etc. It would not be an exaggeration to say that many of my students have spent roughly $1500 to take a two-day course. When that kind of money is being spent, it's fairly easy for me to say, "Hey, that gun doesn't fit your hand, get one that does." Losing $100 in a trade or having to spend an extra $50 for a holster is a small price to pay for huge gains in efficiency. But when I get military personnel sent to me and they are carrying the gun they were issued and it doesn't fit their hand, we work around it to find solutions.

Physical comfort is also important in a class. You must be able to do whatever it is I'm teaching you to do, and if your gun doesn't fit your hand it will affect how well you can perform the skills you are trying to learn. In extreme cases, it makes some skills impossible to accomplish.

I've addressed fit in regard to the strong side and the back of the gun, now I want to examine the weak side. First and foremost, I don't recommend any firearm that has extra levers or buttons beyond the trigger, a slide lock lever and a magazine release. If your gun has a manually operated external safety, or if your gun has a de-cocker, it's not the most efficient style of gun that is available for your personal defense or your armed professional use at this point in time. I'm an advocate for modern striker fired guns. If you're not carrying a modern striker fired gun for personal defense, there needs to be a very good, compelling reason why you would be carrying a gun that is inherently more complicated, and therefore, less efficient. It takes more time, effort, and energy to learn how to proficiently use a more complicated gun. There are more opportunities for failure when you're using a more complicated gun in an ambush moment. It also requires finer motor skills (even extra motor skills), and that sets you up for more potential failure in a counter ambush moment.

Hopefully the only buttons or levers you will need to worry about using regularly are the trigger and the magazine release. You want to make sure that the firearm fits in your hand so that you can use the trigger properly, and that you can hit the magazine release efficiently when reloading. Personally, though I shoot Glocks more often than any other gun, I cannot hit the magazine release conveniently. Because of this, I generally install an extended magazine release on my Glocks. The extended/oversized magazine releases are one of the few modifications to defensive guns that are often a good idea. Ensuring that your trigger finger can touch the trigger and that your thumb can hit the magazine release without changing your grip on the gun are very important components of fit to your handgun. If you find a gun that fits you well for shooting and requires only minimal movement of the hand around the gun to release the magazine during a reload, you can often develop a method for making that movement without losing any time on your reload. If you are forced to make a gross change in the position of your grip or use your weak hand to release the magazine, you should change guns.

The other lever that you will find on most modern defensive and striker-fired guns is a slide-lock (or, on older guns, a slide release) lever. This lever allows you to pull the slide back and lock the gun open (This function is for the purposes of clearing a malfunction, cleaning, putting it away, etc.). Again, it is best if you can do this without shifting your grip.

There are three things that are necessary in order for your defensive gun to be a good fit: you must be able to actuate the trigger, actuate the magazine release, and actuate the slide lock if you need to during a malfunction exercise. If you can't do those three things with a particular gun, then the gun does not fit your hand. If you happen to be stuck with a gun that has extra levers or buttons, you still want to be able to use them with little or no change of your hand position on the gun even though the extra buttons or levers may not be ideal. Being able to run either a safety lever or a de-cocker with your strong hand thumb without shifting your grip is important for your efficiency and consistency.

There are several different types and brands of guns in the modern striker fired gun category that don't have any extra levers or buttons. Which one you choose is largely going to be based on your personal preference, budget, and which one actually fits your hand the best in terms of the width, girth, and the length of the pull of the trigger.

In Memory of Michael DeBose

I offer this separate dedication on a very deep and personal level to former Ohio State Representative, Michael DeBose from Cleveland, Ohio and his family. Rep. DeBose's story appeared as the chapter, *The Political Bravery of Michael DeBose* in *Lessons from Armed America*, with Kathy Jackson. He had voted against Ohio's Concealed Carry legislation twice before changing his mind about armed self-defense and subsequently changing his vote in favor after becoming a victim of an armed assault while strolling through his neighborhood on an afternoon walk. I reached out to him after reading his story in the *Cleveland Plain Dealer* and he granted me an extensive interview. He wanted his story in print and later would became a vocal and public advocate for the right to bear arms, challenging his own party line. The two of us developed a unique bond and a quick friendship that saw him calling me "just to say hello", to wish my family a "happy Thanksgiving, or seek advice on a choice of carry gun. Representative Michael DeBose passed away on April 23, 2012 of complications from Parkinson's disease at the young age of 58. Although it took a life-threatening experience for him to understand the right to bear arms for self-defense, Michael DeBose exhibited incredible strength and courage standing up to the political forces within the vehemently anti-gun forces of his own party and a rabidly anti-gun local media. He is evidence that the right to bear arms knows no boundaries, be they political, racial or economic and that we all share the basic human right to defend our lives. He is missed.

– Mark Walters

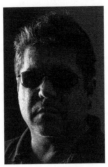

Mark Walters is the nationally syndicated host of the Armed American Radio broadcast distributed by Salem Radio Network and co-author of "Lessons from Armed America" with Kathy Jackson. Mark's regular column, "One to the Head" can be read in the Delta Defense, LLC publication, Concealed Carry Magazine. Mark has discussed the right to bear arms as a guest on national television programs as well as too many local and national radio broadcasts to count. He has appeared as a guest speaker on the subject at several venues including the Second Amendment March in Washington, D.C. and the Gun Rights Policy Conference. Mark can be reached at aarradio@gmail.com

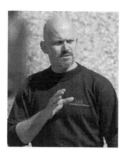

Rob Pincus is a teacher who has been active in the firearms and personal defense industry for over 20 years. He owns and operates I.C.E. Training Company and is the developer of the Combat Focus® Shooting Program. He has produced over 75 Training DVDs with Personal Defense Network™, written several other books including *Combat Focus Shooting: Evolution 2010* and *Counter Ambush* and taught courses at scores of locations across the United States and Europe.

Made in the USA
San Bernardino, CA
04 December 2014